Sandra Cabot MD

I can't lose weight!
...and I don't know why

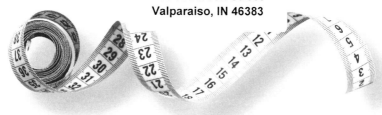

This is the ONLY book that explains
ALL the hidden causes of weight excess!

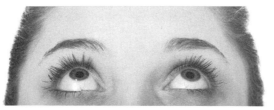

Published in USA by

SCB International
2027 W Rose Garden Lane Phoenix, AZ 85027
Ph +1 623 334 3232

www.liverdoctor.com
www.sandracabot.com
www.drsandracabotclinics.com.au

© 2015 Sandra Cabot MD
ISBN 978-1-936609-32-1

HEA048000	HEALTH & FITNESS / Diet & Nutrition / General
HEA019000	HEALTH & FITNESS / Diet & Nutrition / Weight Loss
HEA006000	HEALTH & FITNESS / Diet & Nutrition / Diets

Categories

1.Weight Control. 2. Weight Loss 3. Syndrome X. 4. Diet 5. Nutrition 6. Diabetes 7. Polycystic Ovarian Syndrome 8. Metabolism 9. Fat Burning 10. Low carbohydrate 11. Paleo eating 12. Metabolic syndrome 13. Insulin resistance

Contents

Contents

Contents

Contents

About the Author

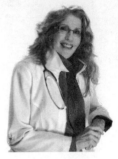 Sandra Cabot MD is a medical doctor who has extensive clinical experience in treating patients with weight problems, chronic medical problems, liver problems and hormonal imbalances. Dr Cabot works with other medical doctors and her team of naturopaths in Sydney Australia and Phoenix Arizona in the USA.

Dr Sandra Cabot began studying nutritional medicine while she was a medical student and has been a pioneer in the area of holistic healing. She graduated in medicine with honors from Adelaide University, South Australia in 1975.

During the early 1980s Dr Cabot worked as a volunteer in the largest missionary Christian hospital in Northern India, tending to the poor indigenous women.

Dr Cabot has written 30 books on health including the award winning Liver Cleansing Diet Book. She is a pilot and is a proud supporter of the Angel Flight Charity.

Introduction

It's a grim statistic: Most people who go on a diet and lose weight end up regaining that weight within a year.

Why does this happen?

There are many reasons why people fail to lose their excess weight with the most common being –

- Stress gets in the way
- They lose their focus
- They lack self belief – whether you think you can or think you can't, you're right

To overcome these obstacles you need to get the right support and tools from the best people. You will find it difficult to achieve your goal of weight loss by yourself because your own mind will try to sabotage you along the way, especially when stress or fatigue comes along. This is when you need to get help to refocus on yourself. You will need ongoing guidance, support and motivation. My team of Weight Loss Detectives (WLDs) can provide all those things and have been trained by me in my weight loss methods. My WLDs are situated in Phoenix Arizona in the USA and Sydney New South Wales in Australia. They can be contacted by phone, skype and email – see page 22

Support groups like Over Eaters Anonymous are also extremely valuable if you go to their meetings regularly.

This book will give you the right knowledge and tools to be successful and I suggest you use it as your weight loss bible and refer to it regularly. Don't hesitate to contact my WLDs if you need help with your weight loss. A big reason that people fail to lose weight is that they view a "diet" as a short-term solution and don't really change their thinking. Our Weight Loss Detective program focuses on REAL sustainable, permanent change. It's not hype!

About this book

If you are battling with a weight problem, this book has a strategy that I truly believe can help you for the rest of your life.

I have an incredible life that has given me the opportunity to communicate face to face with hundreds of thousands of men and women. Most of these people come to see me looking for help with their weight and hormonal problems.

My organization receives hundreds of E-mails daily from people all over the world. Some people may find this daunting but I find it fascinating and challenging. This is because my weight loss strategies are able to offer these people a healthy and lasting solution to their problems. These people have tried many different things to overcome their weight problems but find that there are missing parts to the jig saw puzzle, which means that they do not know where to start. They will often relate how they have tried every possible diet on the market and taken every type of diet pill, but still continue to gain weight. They feel extremely frustrated, disappointed and confused.

The major obstacle is that they lack a plan or strategy that is tailor made for them, and takes into account **all the reasons that prevent them from losing weight.**

After 40 years of medical research and clinical practice I have been able to focus on the hidden problems that prevent people from losing weight. I have also developed new treatments that can overcome these medical problems safely and naturally. They will work for you, as they scientifically attack the medical problems that cause your metabolism to be abnormal. My approach works on the causes of weight excess, which means that if you can adopt my program as a lifestyle, you will gradually be successful.

If you are overweight you need to recognize the underlying problems that are keeping you fat. If you do not understand the enemy you cannot fight the battle and win. The 12 week Metabolic Weight Loss Plan in this book and my team of

Weight Loss Detectives provide the best strategy for you to win.

> *People believe they are fat just because they eat too much, don't exercise enough or have inherited the wrong genes from their parents. This is a far too simplistic and limited attitude. Indeed these people are very surprised and often relieved to learn that they have several medical problems that may be making them fat.*

When a patient with a weight problem consults one of our Weight Loss Detectives we check -

- Do they suffer with Syndrome X?
- Do they have a dysfunctional or fatty liver?
- Do they have imbalances in their sex hormones?
- Do they have leptin resistance?
- Do they have a thyroid gland problem?
- Do they have an overload of toxins?
- Do they have food intolerances and/or food allergies?
- Do they have the wrong balance of bacteria in their intestines?
- Do they have fluid retention due to sluggish kidneys?
- Do they have impaired metabolism?
- Do they have imbalances in their brain chemicals (neurotransmitters)?
- Do they have a sleeping disorder?
- Do they have a negative belief pattern?

Only after **all the above factors** are taken into account can a tailor made strategy for their own individual weight problem be developed and fine tuned over time. I think this makes a lot of sense, don't you?

I am sure you know people who seem to overeat, but manage to stay slim, and others who seem to eat very little, but remain overweight. This is because body weight and body shape are greatly affected by genetic, metabolic, hormonal and psychological factors, and not just by how much a person eats every day. What we eat is often more important than how much we eat. This is because the molecules in different foods will affect our genes, liver and gut function, and our brain chemistry, and this will impact on metabolism and hormonal balance.

Do not worry that because this book takes into account ALL the factors that could be keeping you overweight, it must therefore be complicated; it is not; indeed it will bring you clarity and direction.

To help you to be successful I have a team of dedicated and qualified people called The Weight Loss Detectives (WLDs) who can support you through the phone, skype and the Internet, and if needed via face to face consults. See page 22

Our websites offer you a wealth of information and I encourage you to visit them and send your questions by email.

The websites are –

> www.liverdoctor.com
> www.sandracabot.com
> www.drsandracabotclinics.com.au

If you need more help phone 623 334 3232 in the USA or 02 4655 8855 in Australia

It can be so confusing

Thirty years ago when I started writing there was a lack of information regarding nutritional medicine and natural therapies. People were starving for information especially about natural therapies, diet and hormones. Today the opposite has happened and people suffer with information overload. Yes there are too many diets, so many supplements and so many philosophies, and in one lifetime you cannot possibly do them all! Furthermore, you cannot try all these things successfully without some form of long term support and direction.

You need to know is what is right for you as an individual

You need to know in your particular case, if there are specific medical problems that are keeping you fat. That is why I have developed The Weight Loss Detective Program where all these factors can be addressed. My team of Weight Loss Detectives are dedicated to your success.

Several years ago I read with amusement, an article published in a medical journal titled *Cardiologist's Fat Fight*. It described the extreme clashing of expert opinions at the annual meeting of the American College of Cardiology. Supporters of the official low fat approach argued with opponents who believed it was excess carbohydrates and not fat that caused weight excess.

The main opponents were the late cardiologist Dr Robert Atkins, and cardiologist Dr Dean Ornish who had totally opposite views on the best diet to prevent obesity caused by Syndrome X.

Dr Atkins promoted his low-carbohydrate, high-fat, high-protein diet, while Dr Ornish promoted a rigorous vegetarian diet low in fat and high in complex carbohydrates. If the experts have totally different approaches and cannot agree, then who can?

I believe that the types of food we eat on a regular basis are crucial to our health and weight control success, and in most of my patients I need to make dietary changes. I find that it is extremely rare to find someone who has a perfect diet, especially bearing in mind that this means different things to different people, including the experts!

It is true that when we look around, people are generally eating less fat and more carbohydrates, and yet they are getting fatter! Indeed some experts believe that a high carbohydrate, low-fat diet can be dangerous to your health and lead to obesity and diabetes.

But I have also found that it is not the diet alone that needs to be considered, but the individual problems that may be sabotaging your best efforts at following a healthy diet, no matter whose diet you follow. Yes we need to look a little deeper into our health in much the same way as a detective would solve a mysterious case. Let us find the missing pieces of the jig saw puzzle so that we can see the overall picture and begin the holistic approach that leaves no stone unturned. Only then are our chances of success very high.

The missing parts to the jig saw puzzle include:

- Syndrome X which is also known as the Metabolic Syndrome or Insulin Resistance
- Leptin resistance – leptin is a hormone that regulates hunger
- Fatty liver or sluggish liver function
- Imbalances in the sex hormones
- Excess cortisol levels caused by stress – cortisol is an adrenal hormone
- Thyroid gland problems such as thyroid resistance and low levels of the thyroid hormone called T 3
- Our genes – this is our unique DNA which we inherit from both parents
- Body toxicity and excess inflammation
- Gut problems such as unhealthy bacteria in the intestines
- Food intolerances and food allergies
- Fluid retention
- A sluggish metabolism
- A chemical imbalance in the brain's neuro-transmitters, especially low dopamine
- A negative self belief pattern

So stay with me and allow me to help you solve your own jig saw puzzle. Read on and discover that what seems at first to be hidden, difficult and confusing, is in fact not hard to understand; knowledge is power and will enable you to overcome your weight problem.

Interesting case histories

During one of my seminars in 1999, I met a woman who really showed me how important it is to consider all the medical reasons that can make a person chronically obese and unwell. Donna was 47 years old and had suffered with polycystic ovaries for many years, which unfortunately had been inadequately treated. Donna was very overweight, and being an Android Body Type (apple shaped) she carried all of her excess weight in her upper body and abdomen. She had lost most of her hair and was almost bald in the male pattern of baldness, although she hid this well with a colored headband over her forehead. She had a fatty liver, Syndrome X and was hypertensive. Although she was almost of menopausal age, she complained of heavy menstrual bleeding, which was due to the deficiency of the hormone progesterone, commonly seen in women who do not ovulate regularly. She was taking the drug Aldactone, in an attempt to reduce her excessive male hormones but this was not controlling her hormonal and metabolic imbalance. Indeed she was going nowhere and had been trapped in a hormonal and metabolic nightmare for years. I thought to myself *"if only I had been able to see this woman 20 years ago, what a difference I could have made to her physical and mental state"*. This woman needed specific help to address ALL of the medical problems that were making her obese and destroying her looks. However it is never too late to restore normal body chemistry and she was still looking for a solution after all these years.

I started her on my dietary program for Syndrome X, and gave her supplements to reduce her high insulin levels and reduce her cravings for carbohydrates. I also stopped the Aldactone, which was not helping her bleeding and hair loss. I prescribed the anti-male hormone medication called Cyproterone acetate, which acts as a type of progesterone to reduce heavy bleeding, and is also very effective at reducing high levels of male hormones.

To be able to balance her metabolism and get her excess weight off, I had to -

- Reverse her chemical imbalance of insulin resistance
- Balance her sex hormones
- Improve her liver function
- Take into account her Body Type

Someone like this presents a real challenge, and needs powerful strategies that look at ALL the imbalances that perpetuate obesity.

Within 6 months I had brought her hormonal problems under control, so that her vaginal bleeding had gone and her hair was growing back. Lowering the male hormones had made it much easier for her to lose the weight from her upper body, as excess male hormones increase insulin resistance and thus fat gain.

It took me 12 months to reverse her fatty liver condition and during this time, as her liver started to burn fat normally, she gradually lost her abdominal obesity. The supplements and liver tonics had also helped her to speed up her sluggish metabolism.

It gave me great satisfaction to see this woman change from an obese masculine balding woman, to an attractive middle aged woman with thicker hair and a normal body weight.

Another interesting case history comes from Dr. Tom Eanelli MD, who is a medical specialist working with cancer patients in New Jersey USA. Dr. Eanelli was suffering with fatty liver, which had caused his weight to balloon to 325 pounds (148kg). He found it impossible to lose weight and was frustrated by the lack of information available on fatty liver condition. One day whilst searching in a book store, he came across my book on the liver titled **The Liver Cleansing Diet**. He read the book and was astounded to learn that his fatty liver could be treated by a specific nutritional program. Dr Eanelli followed the eating plan and took Livatone liver tonic every day. Gradually over a two year period he was able to reverse his fatty liver and got down to 185 pounds (84Kg). Dr Eanelli believes that I saved his life, which is true, as a fatty liver is a serious condition. His case history demonstrates dramatically how essential it is to treat the medical causes of obesity if one is to achieve long lasting success. Dr Eanelli was so inspired by his results that he co-authored a book with me titled *Fatty Liver – You Can Reverse It.*

How to use this book

For those who want to get started straight away, turn to page 34 and start reading!

This section contains the 12-Week Metabolic Weight Loss Plan. Simply start following the easy menus/recipes and begin to re-direct your metabolism from fat-storing into fat-burning straight away.

You can then use the Table of Contents to choose the subjects that interest you.

If you have questions, feel free to call our help-line on 623 334 3232 in the USA or 02 4655 8855 in Australia to speak to a naturopath or email ehelp@liverdoctor.com

Why can't I burn fat?

It's all to do with insulin

The hormone insulin is made in the pancreas gland, and is secreted into the blood stream from the pancreas in response to a rise in blood sugar (glucose). After circulating in the blood stream for only 6 to 10 minutes, the insulin binds with specific receptors on the cell membranes to transfer glucose from the blood stream into the cells. The hormone insulin is extremely powerful and controls the processing of blood glucose.

Everything you eat and drink is absorbed from the small intestine and passes into the portal vein, which takes the nutrients straight to the liver. Fats are broken down into glycerol and fatty acids, while protein is broken down into amino acids, and the liver processes all these nutrients. Carbohydrates are absorbed from the gut as simple sugars, which quickly become glucose in the blood.

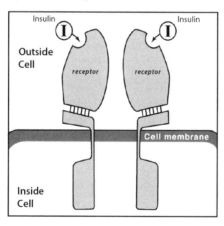

The insulin receptor straddles the cell membrane and

allows sugar to be transported inside the cell.

If you eat a lot of carbohydrate, this will produce a lot of glucose in your blood stream. Glucose is pure energy, and your body has to decide how much of this glucose it will use for immediate energy needs, and how much glucose it will store for future energy needs. It is the powerful hormone insulin, which makes this decision and sends the glucose to the areas of your body that are most suitable and accessible. After a meal, as the blood glucose rises, the pancreas pumps out insulin, which converts some of the blood glucose into a starch called glycogen, which is stored in the muscle and liver cells for future use. Once the glycogen stores are full, excess blood glucose will be converted by the insulin into fat, which is called triglyceride. This triglyceride can be carried in your blood stream to the fatty tissues where it will be deposited as more fat. So we could say that insulin encourages the storage of fat, and that is why **insulin has been called the fat producing hormone.**

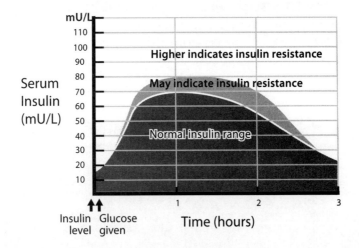

Blood insulin levels

If there is not enough insulin, as in type 1 diabetics, the blood glucose cannot be transferred into glycogen or fat, and the levels of blood glucose rise to dangerously high levels. If there is too much insulin, the blood glucose levels become unstable and may fluctuate from too high to too low. If blood sugar levels fall to dangerously low levels, so that there is not enough sugar to fuel the brain, this sends emergency signals to your hormonal system, which responds by pumping out hormones such as adrenalin (epinephrine), cortisol and glucagon to liberate glucose urgently into the blood stream.

The types of foods in your diet will have a big effect upon the amount of insulin that you have in your blood stream. If you eat meals that are high in refined carbohydrates, such as flour and sugar, the blood glucose will rise rapidly causing a rapid increase in insulin levels. Conversely meals containing mostly fat and protein, but low in carbohydrates, do not cause a large rise in blood glucose, and therefore do not require much insulin to be processed. Protein foods require only a small amount of insulin, whereas fat requires virtually no insulin to process.

Metabolic Imbalance

Metabolic imbalance is caused by Syndrome X and is a problem with the metabolism of sugar and fat. Syndrome X is also known as metabolic resistance or the metabolic syndrome.

The X factor was hidden and mysterious, until Professor Gerald Reaven first described it in 1988. He named it *Syndrome X* because it was largely unknown and not recognized at this time as being a significant factor in the genesis of disease and obesity.

Today, insulin resistance is widely recognized by the medical profession as a forerunner to heart disease and type 2 diabetes; but unfortunately insulin resistance is still greatly underestimated as a cause of obesity.

Insulin resistance is caused by a disturbance in the function of the hormone insulin, which is really the root cause of the problem. In insulin resistance the body becomes resistant to the action of insulin and to compensate, the pancreas over produces insulin. This disturbance of insulin function leads to all the symptoms of Syndrome X. This can be compared to a builder who has hired workers to build a house. If the workers are inefficient or lazy, the builder has to hire more workers to compensate for the inefficient workers; otherwise the work will never be completed on time. This is what happens in your body if you have Syndrome X – your insulin is lazy and inefficient and to compensate your pancreas has to make a lot more insulin. You end up with way too much insulin.

I describe Syndrome X as the chemical imbalance that makes you fat. Syndrome X is the most common and potent medical reason why people cannot lose weight. Indeed Syndrome X makes it virtually impossible to lose weight unless it is specifically treated.

Syndrome X is a collection of symptoms and medical signs which may include:

- Insulin resistance (the body's cells do not respond to insulin)
- High blood levels of the hormone insulin
- Weight excess especially in the abdominal area
- Fatty liver
- Cravings for carbohydrates
- Excess hunger
- Abnormalities in blood fats
- A variety of blood glucose abnormalities
- High blood levels of uric acid may be present
- High blood pressure may be present
- Fatigue because carbohydrates are not being burnt for energy but are stored as fat

Professor Reaven's research team first recognized that people with insulin resistance have an elevated risk of diabetes and heart disease. Reaven also found that a high carbohydrate diet could raise the insulin levels and thus the risk of heart disease. Although Syndrome X is usually associated with weight excess, it can also be found in non-obese, non-diabetic persons if they have a poor diet.

Insulin Resistance

This term means that the body is resistant to the effects of the hormone insulin, so that your body has lost the ability to respond to the insulin. Your body cells resist the insulin, so that the pancreas has to secrete more insulin to make up for this lack of sensitivity. In those with insulin resistance the insulin is not able to transfer glucose from the blood into the cells very efficiently. This causes the blood glucose levels to gradually rise over the years.

The resistance to insulin results from defects in the sensitivity of the body cells to insulin. The body cells become insensitive to insulin because the receptors on the surface of the cells do not communicate efficiently with the insulin.

It is as if the receptors become accustomed to the high insulin levels and become desensitized to them - it's like the boy who cried wolf and in the end no one took him seriously.

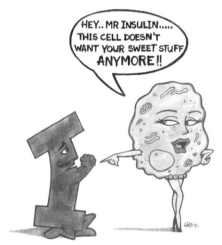

Yes the snobby cells just ignore the insulin!

What causes Insulin Resistance (IR)?

In modern day industrialized societies around 40% of the population is unable to metabolize carbohydrates efficiently. This is due to a combination of genetics, processed foods, excess carbohydrate intake and a lack of exercise.

Weight excess can cause insulin resistance (IR), and resistance to the action of insulin is a characteristic feature of human obesity. It is the ingestion of too much refined carbohydrate that triggers the release of high levels of insulin, but the body cells cannot respond to this insulin. In insulin resistance (IR) the insulin becomes less and less effective at converting glucose into cellular energy, and more of this glucose is transferred into fat deposits. We find that high levels of insulin and IR occur in the vast majority of overweight people.

In those with IR, although the insulin cannot get glucose into the cells efficiently, it can still perform other functions such as –

- Converting carbohydrates into body fat and fat in the liver
- Suppressing the burning of stored fat

In a person with normal metabolism, around 40% of dietary carbohydrate is converted into fat, whereas in a person with IR, that percentage is much higher. People with IR are not designed to eat the amount of carbohydrates found in the modern day diet of wealthy developed countries.

In people with normal insulin metabolism the body cells are **not** resistant to the action of insulin and only small amounts of insulin are required to control the blood glucose levels. These people do not battle with their weight, as excess quantities of the fat producing hormone insulin are not produced. Their blood glucose levels are generally more stable, so that they do not get the strong cravings for carbohydrates so typical of those with IR. These people are designed to be able to eat more carbohydrates without metabolic problems.

In those with IR, symptoms such as fatigue, mental fogginess, mood changes, shakiness and insatiable hunger for carbohydrates frequently occur. This is because the glucose is not getting inside the cells so that the cells are not able to produce adequate energy. Thus you don't have the energy to exercise, which makes it harder to lose the weight.

In IR, there may also be a delayed responsiveness of your cells to insulin, so that at first the high amounts of insulin do not work. Eventually some hours after eating, the insulin starts to work, causing a large drop in blood glucose, so you suffer with hypoglycemia. Hypoglycemia makes you extremely tired and unable to function mentally or physically. This causes a sudden urge to eat more carbohydrates, which will then send up the insulin levels again, so that the glucose is converted to fat.

You feel trapped in a vicious cycle believing that it is your will power that is at fault. Well, stop feeling guilty, because you are a victim of a chemical imbalance.

You are locked into a metabolic problem that is making you fatter and fatter!

High levels of the hormone insulin

In Syndrome X the blood insulin levels become elevated because the body needs higher and higher amounts of insulin to control the blood glucose levels.

High levels of insulin are damaging to your health for several reasons -

- They cause a derangement of fat metabolism – namely the blood fats called triglyceride and the bad (LDL) cholesterol increases and the good cholesterol (HDL) levels go down
- They increase the development of fatty plaques in your arteries (atherosclerosis)
- They cause a fatty liver

- They increase the retention of salt and water and stimulate the growth of smooth muscle cells in the arteries, which elevates blood pressure.
- They may affect the brain chemicals (neuro-transmitters), causing mood disorders and insomnia
- They **suppress** the levels of two important slimming hormones in your body -

  - Glucagon - which promotes the burning of sugar and fat

  - Growth hormone - which is needed for building new muscle mass

- They promote the conversion of blood glucose into triglyceride fats and thus encourage fat deposits in your body - **in other words insulin tends to make you fat**.

You can see that **high levels of insulin increase the risk factors for cardiovascular disease**. Because obesity and high insulin levels usually go together, explains why being overweight is a major risk factor for your heart. If we can stop the vicious cycle of insulin resistance and high insulin levels, you will not only have a powerful weapon to lose weight, you will also be able to reduce your risk of heart disease and diabetes and increase your life span.

Syndrome X is very common, and may be seen in as many as one in three persons, or 33% of a normal non-diabetic population. *(REF. 1)*

If the chemical imbalance of Syndrome X is allowed to continue it can result in diabetes. Diabetes occurs when the cells are so resistant to insulin, that the blood glucose continues to rise to abnormally high levels and remains continuously elevated. Diabetes is extremely common in overweight people and there is now an epidemic of diabetes in wealthy countries.

Eventually the insulin production may become inadequate because the insulin producing cells in the pancreas are exhausted. The pancreas becomes worn out and is unable to keep on producing the huge amount of insulin that is required to control the blood glucose levels. This is called pancreatic burnout and it is then necessary to prescribe insulin therapy. This is how a type 2 diabetic turns into a type 1 diabetic who now requires insulin.

Why is Syndrome X often missed?

Syndrome X is often not handled correctly because there is a tendency to treat the symptoms of this chemical imbalance, rather than attack the cause of insulin resistance. Those with Syndrome X are often on multiple drugs such as cholesterol lowering drugs, blood thinners, antihypertensive drugs and blood sugar lowering drugs – just imagine how hard their fatty liver has to work to break down all these drugs? Overworking the liver like this often leads to weight gain because all the liver's energy is used up to breakdown the drugs and there is less liver energy to burn fat– wow what a vicious circle we can create if we only treat the symptoms!

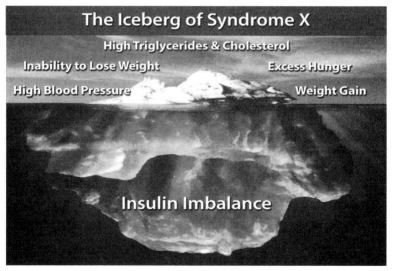

The Iceberg of Syndrome X
High Triglycerides & Cholesterol
Inability to Lose Weight   Excess Hunger
High Blood Pressure   Weight Gain

Insulin Imbalance

Some researchers have compared Syndrome X to an iceberg with its cause hidden beneath the surface of the ocean. At the top of the iceberg we see only the peaks of ice, which represent the symptoms. The symptoms we may see are obesity, abnormal blood fats, raised blood pressure and disturbances of blood glucose levels. Doctors treat these symptoms with drugs, which may be needed but hopefully not forever, if we are able to correct the insulin disturbance, which is the cause of these symptoms.

Excess body fat is a symptom of Syndrome X, and is usually treated with a low-fat diet. However this type of diet does not lower the raised insulin level, which is the cause of the obesity. We need an eating plan and supplement program to normalize the insulin metabolism. Only then are we able to overcome the obesity and all the other symptoms of Syndrome X.

Not only is Syndrome X the leading medical cause of obesity, it is also a leading cause of cardiovascular disease.

Abdominal obesity

If you carry excess body fat in the abdominal area, and find it very difficult to lose the weight there is a very high chance that you have Syndrome X. Insulin has a much stronger effect upon fat cells in the abdominal area, and high levels of insulin will cause fat storage most easily in the abdomen and upper body. Abdominal obesity is associated with high levels of insulin, and therefore with all the other risks of high insulin, such as abnormal blood fats, high blood pressure and a predilection to heart disease and diabetes.

Where you carry your excess body fat is even more important for your health than your total weight. If you store excess weight in the abdominal area it is important to understand where this excess fat is laid down. The excess fat not only accumulates underneath the skin of the abdominal wall, but also inside the abdominal cavity and around your body organs. In the early stages, the fat accumulates around the liver, stomach, pancreas, intestines and kidneys. As Syndrome X progresses, the increasing fat begins to accumulate around the heart, and starts to infiltrate or invade the body organs, so you may develop a fatty pancreas or worst of all a fatty liver.

Abdominal obesity is more common in men and in Android (apple-shaped) women, but can eventually occur in anyone with Syndrome X, if fat accumulation continues unabated.

High levels of insulin can promote storage of excess fat anywhere in the body. However if you carry most of your excess fat around your buttocks, hips and thighs, and not around your abdomen, you will be less likely to develop the higher risk of heart disease and diabetes that comes with abdominal obesity. This is because in the hip and thigh areas, there are no body cavities or vital organs that can be infiltrated with fat. The excess fat accumulates only in the layers between the muscles and skin, and often produces a marbled or cellulite appearance to the surface of the buttocks, hips and thighs. If the pear shaped (gynaeoid) woman continues to gain body fat, her excess fat may eventually accumulate in the abdominal area, and she will become a victim of Syndrome X. It is not uncommon to find that pear shaped women who have carried excess weight in the thigh/hip area for years, without any metabolic problems, suddenly put on a lot of weight in the abdominal area during the peri-menopausal years.

The 12-week Metabolic Weight Loss Plan

Stage One

Stage One consists of eight weeks of very low carbohydrate intake

Stage one is a very important stage so really try to focus and follow stage one exactly with no variations. This is because it takes around 8 weeks to redirect your metabolism from being a sugar burner into a fat burner. After this time your hunger hormones (insulin and leptin) and the appetite center in your brain have been rebooted. You will feel much better and quite different. After these 8 weeks you will not be as tired and cravings for the wrong foods will disappear.

If you do stray and eat high carbohydrate foods during stage one, exercise it off. This will keep your insulin levels down. You may decide to start again at the beginning of the 8 weeks, or just add the days or weeks at the end of the 8 weeks, during which you could not follow the diet.

Food choices during the first 8 weeks

During these 8 weeks you can choose ONLY the recipes in this book that are marked with stage one. These recipes are lower in carbohydrate and higher in protein.

You will NOT be able to eat any of the following - bread, pasta, rice, noodles, cereals, cakes, biscuits, crackers, muffins, pastries, candies, chocolate, sugar, sweet drinks, soft drinks, desserts or starchy vegetables (potatoes, pumpkin, parsnip or swede).

You will be more successful if you choose the low carbohydrate vegetables and the low carbohydrate green leafy salads, accompanied by pure protein such as eggs, cheese, plain yoghurt, seafood and fresh meat.

If you are a vegan choose legumes instead of grains during stage one. It is harder for a vegan who eats no animal protein at all to get their insulin levels low so they can burn fat. Animal protein such as dairy, eggs, poultry and meat and seafood is much lower in carbohydrates than vegetarian foods

You may use healthy fats such as cold pressed olive and nut oils, coconut oil, tahini, avocado, raw nuts and seeds and even some butter !

You can have legumes, but be aware that although they have a low GI, they contain significant amounts of carbohydrate, although less than grains. If you like legumes, you may eat them in very small amounts (½ cup twice a week) during stage one. Lentils are the best choice of legumes for weight loss. Some people however are unable to eat any legumes, as they may cause indigestion, gas and pain symptoms. People with autoimmune diseases may find that legumes and grains aggravate their inflammation.

You can have 2 serves of fresh fruits daily, but no more, and avoid the fruits higher in sugar such as banana, mango, figs, grapes and papaya during stage one. Avoid dried fruits. The best fruits for weight loss are citrus, passion fruit, berries, prunes and green apples.

If you use milk of any kind in your tea and coffee make sure that it does not contain any sugar; note that many brands of soy milk contain sugar.

How much weight will I lose during stage one?

Your weight loss will vary, according to -

- The state of your liver
- Your insulin and leptin levels – if they are very high it takes longer to get them down
- The accuracy with which you follow the Weight Loss Plan
- The amount of exercise you do

Most people can expect a weekly weight loss of one to two

pounds (½ to 1 kilogram), while in others the rate of weight loss may be much more than this.

Do NOT focus on the amount of weight you are losing, as your mind will use this to sabotage you. Instead concentrate on following the recipes and menus exactly and making time for exercise. Some people have an obsession with weighing themselves and use slow weight loss as an excuse to give up – if you are one of these types, remove the scales from your home.

There will be some of you who will benefit by staying on stage one for longer than 8 weeks –

- If you have a fatty liver
- If you have been overweight for many years
- If you have been a chronic yo-yo dieter
- If you are an overweight diabetic
- If you have more than 20 kilograms (44 pounds) of weight to lose

Please be patient, as if you have a fatty liver, it can take 6 to 12 months to reverse this condition.

It is quite safe to stay on stage one for as long as you like! Many people choose to stay on stage one for 16 weeks or longer or even adopt it as their permanent way of eating

For those who want more rapid weight loss-

I suggest that you follow a very low carbohydrate diet (say less than 20 to 40grams of carbohydrate daily), under the supervision of your health care professional or one of my WLDs. This is known as a Ketogenic Diet and it always works. See page 305 for the Ketogenic Diet

If you want a Weight Loss Detective to guide you on a Ketogenic Diet contact our Australian office on 02 4655 8855 or email ehelp@liverdoctor.com

Stage Two

The Second Stage consists of four weeks of low carbohydrate intake

During these 4 weeks you are able to use only the recipes marked with Stage 2 and Stage 1. However you should limit desserts to two per week.

You will be allowed to have one slice of bread daily or one serving of starchy vegetables daily.

You can have 2 to 3 serves of fresh fruit daily, but avoid papaya, mangos, bananas and dried fruit.

You can replace the one slice of bread with an extra serve of starchy vegetables, pasta, or a grain such as brown rice if desired.

You can begin the maintenance program, which is Stage Three, once you have reached your desired weight. You can extend Stage 2 if you need to lose more weight.

Stage Three

Stage Three is the Maintenance Plan and can be followed as a general guide for the rest of your life

Stage three provides approximately 40 percent of daily calories from carbohydrate.

You can use any of the recipes in this book and may have 3 desserts a week.

You can have 2 to 3 serves of any fresh fruit daily.

You are allowed to have –
- 2 slices of bread and one serve of starchy vegetables daily
        or
- 1 slice of bread and two serves of starchy vegetables daily
        or

You can replace the 2 slices of bread with 1 serve of pasta or 1 serve of noodles, or more starchy vegetables or 1 serve of a grain such as brown rice.

If you are unable to exercise, you may not be able to eat this much carbohydrate without gaining weight.

The Grain Free Diet

Some people are intolerant to gluten and will find that eating gluten keeps them overweight. Gluten is found in wheat, rye, barley and some types of oats. You do not have to be a celiac to suffer from gluten intolerance. Many people find that any type of bread (even gluten free bread) really slows down their metabolism and clogs up their bowels. In such cases it is better to avoid bread altogether, as it is not necessary for good health and can be the biggest reason you cannot lose weight.

Bread can always be replaced with vegetables. Many people do better with weight loss if they avoid all foods containing wheat, rye, barley, oats and rice; in other words if they have a grain free diet and this is perfectly healthy to follow long term. People with Syndrome X are carbohydrate intolerant and unless they do a lot of exercise they cannot tolerate the carbohydrates that come from grains or sugar. For some people the fact that they continue to eat grains is the biggest reason they cannot lose weight.

Recommended supplements during the 12-Week Metabolic Weight Loss Plan are-

- Glicemic Balance Capsules - 1 capsule three times daily or 2 capsules twice daily to lower insulin levels
- LivaTone Plus - 2 capsules twice daily to increase fat burning in the liver
- Metabocel tablets may be considered if you have a really slow or sluggish metabolism. Metabocel contains the herb Garcinia and other fat burning nutrients
- Syndrome X Slimming Protein Powder for smoothies

Extra Tips

Free Foods

Salad vegetables and green vegetables are free foods, and you may eat as much of these as you like.

For those who are short of time and money you can make any of your meals from -

Canned seafood, eggs, fresh meats, sugar free protein powder (such as whey protein or Synd-X Slimming Protein Powder), canned sugar free or cooked legumes, unprocessed cheeses (such as feta, ricotta, cottage, mature cheese such as parmesan), our high protein bean salad recipes (see page 58), homemade muesli (see page 47), and plenty of fresh salads and vegetables. If you are short of money, you may purchase the baking or loose nuts in the supermarkets, as these are generally cheaper. Remember every time you eat protein make sure you add some fibrous fruits or vegetables to prevent constipation. Remember every time you eat carbohydrate try to include some protein, as this will reduce the rise in blood glucose levels after eating. Boil 6 eggs at a time, so they are ready in the fridge for you to have a snack. Eggs are very healthy, as well as slimming, as they are good for the liver and are very low in carbohydrate

Foods to boost a sluggish metabolism

Many of the recipes in this book contain natural herbs, vegetables and spices that are able to increase the metabolic rate; they are commonly used in Asian cuisine.

Examples of these include -

Garlic, onion, chili, curry, ginger, lime leaves, lemon grass, garam masala, tandoori paste, tamarind paste, coriander, dill, basil, mint, turmeric, cumin, cardamom, cinnamon, cloves, nutmeg, paprika, black pepper and others. We have included these spices and herbs, as research has shown that spicy food and natural herbs are able to speed up the metabolic rate, which is useful for those who are metabolically resistant and do not burn fat easily. Furthermore these natural ingredients add wonderful new and often exotic flavors to the meals, and are excellent substitutes for processed sauces, which are often full of sugar, preservatives and colorings. So do not be surprised to find that you start to lose weight more easily when you include these natural herbs and spices in your meals. For those who do not like the taste or effect of spicy food, it is not a problem to exclude them, as the balance of the food groups in our recipes will still ensure that your metabolism is improved.

Acidic substances help with weight loss

Acidic substances such as vinegar and freshly squeezed lemon, lime and grapefruit juice have a beneficial effect upon the metabolism. They also help the digestive process when they are consumed with a meal. It has been found that the acid content in tart tasting foods, such as vinegar and lemon, can help to moderate the blood glucose elevation that follows the ingestion of carbohydrates; so it is good to include these things with a meal. Organic apple cider vinegar with the mother tincture, which makes it look cloudy instead of clear, is the best vinegar of all to use regularly. This type of apple cider vinegar can be used as part of a salad dressing. Furthermore 1 to 2 tablespoons of organic apple cider vinegar can be drunk in the middle of every meal to assist with weight loss. Don't take it on an empty stomach and some people need to dilute the vinegar with water to avoid it causing stomach discomfort. Those who suffer with poor digestion or those who are taking antacid medications, will benefit greatly from slowly sipping a small glass of water containing 2 tablespoons of apple cider vinegar during a meal. I have had patients who have lost a lot of weight by drinking 2 tablespoons of apple cider vinegar during their meals. This works because it stimulates digestion, improves bacterial flora in the gut and lowers insulin levels after the meal.

How much is one serving of carbohydrate?

4 small cracker biscuits

½ cup cooked pasta, cooked cereal or cooked rice

1 cup cooked legumes

1 cup raw muesli

1 slice of bread

1 sweet biscuit

3 cups raw leafy vegetables

1 cup cooked mixed starchy vegetables

½ cup cooked potatoes

1 cup vegetable juice

1 piece fresh fruit

¼ cup dried fruit (only to be eaten very occasionally). Fresh fruit is far better for weight loss.

You can interchange these servings.

Recipes

Breakfast Recipes

Omelette (Stage 1)

Use any combination of vegetables, herbs and/or meat that you enjoy – such as bacon, chicken, salmon, tuna, broccoli, finely chopped spinach, mushrooms, onion, chives, parsley, garlic, chili, bell peppers (capsicum), cilantro (coriander), rosemary, tomatoes (fresh or sun-dried and chopped), black pepper and sea salt to taste. You may also add 2 tbsp of grated parmesan cheese.

Method: Combine 2 to 3 eggs in a bowl and whisk, add all the other chopped ingredients and mix. Pour into fry pan on a low to medium heat. Then flip mixture in the pan to cook the topside, or place pan under the grill to cook the top of the omelette.

Serves one person

Poached Eggs (Stage 1)

2 to 3 eggs poached. Serve with steamed asparagus and/or some grilled vegetables of your choice.

A freshly made mixed raw vegetable juice or citrus juice made with orange, grapefruit and lemon or lime. Serves one person.

Scrambled Eggs (Stage 1)

2 to 3 eggs scrambled in a pan with unsweetened milk. Season with fresh herbs, pepper and salt. You may serve with cooked thinly sliced mushrooms and chopped chives or grilled tomato halves.

One piece fresh fruit or a mixed raw vegetable juice or one glass tomato juice. — *Serves one person.*

Hard Boiled Eggs   (Stage 1)

2 or 3   Eggs, hard boiled and chopped
¼ cup   Carrot, grated
½ cup   Mixed fresh herbs, chopped (parsley, oregano and mint is a good mix).

Toss together with a little cracked black pepper and 1 teaspoon chili sauce (sweetened with a pinch of stevia powder or some Nature Sweet Sugar Substitute). Alternatively you can mix the hard boiled eggs with curry powder and some salt.

Serve with 2 to 3 olives on the side with a handful of fresh sprouts.

Serves one person.

Grilled Lamb Chops   (Stage 1)

2   Lamb chops

Place chops under the griller. Serve with one tomato (halved) and other vegetables of choice (such as mushrooms, eggplant, bell pepper, asparagus etc.), which can be lightly fried in olive oil or grilled. Add salad vegetables if desired.

Serves one person.

Lean Steak   (Stage 1)

1   Steak, grilled or pan cooked

You may add an egg to grill or poach with this

Serve with grilled or lightly fried vegetables such as tomato, chopped chives, mushrooms, onions and bell peppers. You can add fresh chili or garlic if desired. Use a small amount of olive oil if you fry the vegetables. Serve with black pepper and sea salt to taste.

One grapefruit.

Serves one person.

Sardines or Other Fish   *(Stage 1)*

Choose canned fish in brine/spring water. Serve with grilled or lightly fried vegetables such as eggplant, tomatoes, spring onions, field mushroom, or a green salad.

A raw vegetable juice or tomato juice.

Serves one or more persons.

Avocado and Salmon   *(Stage 1)*

1   Avocado peeled and chopped

1   Slice of fresh pineapple

¼ cup Almonds, chopped or any other chopped fresh nuts

Chop fruit, toss with nuts and sprinkle with 2 tablespoon chopped mint. Gently fold in the contents of a 120 gm (4oz) tin of pink salmon in brine (or tuna in brine).

Serves 2 people.

Herrings or Kippers   *(Stage 1)*

Choose canned or frozen fish. Top with chopped spring onions and chopped parsley or cilantro (coriander), 4 olives and a handful of fresh bean sprouts and a generous squeeze of lemon juice and olive oil to taste.

Can serve hot or cold

One grapefruit.

Serves one person.

Fish Fillet - Fresh or Frozen   *(Stage 1)*

1 large   Fish Fillet or 2 small fillets

Steam or fry fish in a fry pan in a small amount of olive oil

Serve with a good squeeze of lemon juice, 2 sticks of celery, a vine ripened tomato and a handful of alfalfa or bean sprouts and black pepper and salt to taste. A little chopped dill gives this a lovely flavor. You can also add chopped spring onion and cumin if you desire for extra flavor and health benefits.

Serves two people.

Protein Smoothie Drink   (Stage 1)

1-2 cups   *Milk – choose dairy milk or sugar free milk alternatives such as unsweetened soy, almond milk or coconut milk.*

2-3 tbsp   *Synd-X Slimming Protein Powder or whey protein powder*

½ cup   *Berries such as strawberries or frozen berries such as blueberries and raspberries*

Mix all ingredients in a blender.

1 tablespoon of LSA or hemp seeds or chia seeds can be added for extra fiber and essential fatty acids

Water can be used instead of milk if preferred

Serves one person.

Bubble and Squeak   (Stage 1)

Left over mashed vegetables, mixed together with 2 eggs, beaten. Add pepper and salt and spices of choice. Form into rounded patties and warm in a fry pan or under griller. Serve with your favorite non-sweetened relish.

Serves one person.

Yogurt and Fresh Fruit Breakfast   (Stage 1)

1 cup   Greek style or plain yogurt (you can use full fat yogurt if you like it, as it is healthy and satisfying). Remember natural healthy fat does not elevate insulin levels. The yogurt you choose must be sugar free; so check labels, as many fruit flavored yogurts contain a lot of sugar.

1 slice	Cantaloupe or papaya
1	Kiwi fruit or ½ cup berries
1	Pear or 1 Apple or 1 Passion fruit

Preparation

Chop fruit into bite size pieces. Serve with yogurt and sprinkle with 1 to 2 tablespoons of Synd-X Protein Powder or LSA, chia seeds or hemp seeds.

Serves one person.

Quick Breakfast Smoothie　　　　(Stage 1)

1 cup Milk – dairy or unsweetened milk alternative such as sugar free soy, almond, or coconut milk. You may use water if preferred.

Fruit	1 kiwi fruit or ¾ cup berries or strawberries
2 tbsp	Synd-X Slimming Protein Powder or whey protein powder
A dash	vanilla essence
1 tbsp	LSA

Process all in blender until smooth. Sprinkle with cinnamon.

Serves one person

Cooked Fruit with Yogurt　　　　(Stage 1)

2	Green apples
1	Pear or 1 stone fruit

Chop fruit and cook in a small amount of water with one cinnamon stick, two cloves and some grated nutmeg. Add one tsp of Nature Sweet Sugar Substitute or a pinch of stevia for sweetness. Sprinkle over some cinnamon and/or LSA or chia seeds if desired. Serve with half a cup of plain full fat yogurt. — *Serves one person.*

Muesli - Low Carb and High Protein (Stage 2)

3 cups	Rolled oats
2 cups	Hemp seeds (no need to grind)
1 cup	Chia seeds (no need to grind)
2 cups	LSA
½ cup	Almonds, chopped or other nuts of choice
½ cup	Pepitas - these are green pumpkin seeds, chopped
½ cup	Shredded coconut, sugarless
½ cup	Sesame seeds, roasted

Preparation

Mix ingredients all together - store in an airtight container in the refrigerator. This muesli mix provides first class protein, which contains all the essential amino acids.

1 Serve = 3 to 4 tbsp of muesli. It can be served with dairy milk or unsweetened sugar free milk alternatives such as soymilk, almond milk, or coconut milk.

You may add 1 cup of fresh fruit or ½ cup Greek style or plain unsweetened yogurt if desired. It is not necessary to use low fat milks or yogurt, unless you prefer the taste.

A large quantity of this muesli recipe can be made and stored in an airtight container. If you leave out the LSA it will keep well in the cupboard if you sticky tape some bay leaves on the inside of the lid. If it contains LSA store it in an airtight container in the refrigerator. You can store the LSA separately in the refrigerator or freezer and add it to muesli when eaten.

Toast   (Stage 2)

One slice of bread, toasted. Choose wholegrain, rye or sourdough or gluten free if you are intolerant to gluten.

Spread with tahini, hummus or nut paste or a little butter. Top with sliced tomato, avocado and/or sardines. Sprinkle with chopped parsley, sea salt and black pepper.

One piece fresh fruit or a mixed raw vegetable juice.

Serves one person.

Legumes (Beans, Chickpeas or Lentils)   (Stage 2)

400 gram (14 ounces) legumes, choose canned or cook them yourself

Heat in a saucepan some olive oil and tomato paste. Add chopped tomatoes, chopped onion, chives or garlic and capsicums (bell peppers) or other vegetables of choice and heat. Add legumes and warm through.

Serve with a hand full of chopped fresh parsley. If desired, sprinkle with one dessertspoon of LSA.

Serves 3 to 4 people.

Soybeans   (Stage 2)

½ cup   Soybeans – freshly cooked or canned

Cook beans until tender and drain. Return beans to the saucepan and add 1 chopped tomato (can use canned), 2 tbsp chopped chives, 1 tbsp fresh chopped basil, 1 large clove garlic minced (optional), 1 chopped red onion. Warm through, season with salt and pepper.

Serve with a handful of alfalfa, bean sprouts or fresh rocket.

Serves one person.

Muesli – High Fibre   (Stage 3)

2 cups	Rolled oats
1 cup	Hemp seeds
½ cup	Chia seeds
2 cups	LSA
1 cup	Rice bran or oat bran
½ cup	Natural sultanas or currants
½ cup	Dried apricots, chopped
½ cup	Almonds, chopped or other nuts of choice
½ cup	Pepitas – these are green pumpkin seeds, chopped
½ cup	Sunflower seeds
¼ cup	Sesame seeds, roasted
¼ cup	Dried coconut, sugarless

Victoria's Breakfast Cookies   (Stage 1)

2	Eggs, whole
½ cup	Synd X protein powder
½ cup	coconut flour
½ cup	freshly milled raw nuts (not peanuts)
½ cup	coconut oil

175 ml (6oz) coconut cream

Additions may include cacao nibs, cinnamon, nutmeg, antioxidant powder (acai, goji, macqui).

Add some coconut water - add slowly until soft drop consistency is reached.

Mix all ingredients to make a smooth batter and drop dessertspoonfuls onto baking tray covered with baking paper, makes approximately 12/tray.

Bake at 180°C (350°F) until base is golden brown and allow to cool on tray. These are high protein and best stored frozen wrapped in parcels of 4, which is sufficient for a sustaining breakfast or lunch.

Victoria's Paleo Breakfast Cookies (Stage 1)

½ cup	freshly milled chia seed
½ cup	pea protein powder – vanilla or chocolate
½ cup	coconut flour
½ cup	coconut oil
¼ cup	hemp seeds

225ml (80z) coconut cream

½ cup freshly milled raw nuts (not peanuts)

Additions may include cacao nibs, cinnamon, nutmeg, antioxidant powder (acai, goji, macqui).

Add some coconut water - add slowly until soft drop consistency is reached. Mix dry ingredients thoroughly, then combine with coconut oil and cream. Add enough coconut water to a make a smooth batter consistency and drop dessertspoonfuls onto baking tray covered with baking paper, makes approximately 12/tray.

Bake at 180°C (350°F) until base is golden brown. Allow to cool on the tray. These are high protein and best stored frozen wrapped in parcels of 4, which is sufficient for a sustaining breakfast or lunch.

Energizing Drinks to Accompany Breakfast Meals

You may enjoy a mixed vegetable juice with your chosen breakfast, or choose one of our smoothie recipes for your breakfast during any stage of the weight loss program.

Remember you are allowed only 2 pieces of fruit daily whilst on stage 2, and only 3 pieces of fruit daily whilst on stage 3, so watch that you don't exceed your daily allowance.

Those on Stage 1 of the eating plan can only have 1 serve of fresh fruit daily. Strawberries, apricots, honeydew melon, oranges, grapefruit, mandarins, berries, plums, cherries and prunes are the lower carbohydrate fruits to choose if possible.

Healthy Beverage Suggestions

Tomato Refresher & Vitamin C Booster (Stage 1)

Juice enough raw tomato and green apple (⅔ tomato and 1/3 apple mixture) to make about 10oz (300 mls) or 1 large cup of juice. Also juice 4 to 6 fresh basil leaves, and 4 fresh mint leaves. For a spicy tang add 2-3 drops of Tabasco sauce and ¼ tsp freshly grated horseradish. Add ¼ of a lemon. This juice will increase the metabolic rate to assist weight loss.

Serves 2

This juice goes well with a 4.4oz (125g) can of sardines, salmon or tuna, flavored with herbs or chili.

Melon Pep - to start your day   *(Stage 1)*

2 slices	Watermelon – leave some of the inner skin on melon
2	Celery stems and tops
4-6	Mint or basil leaves

Process all in a juicer.

Serve with 1 to 2 lean grilled chops, a small piece of grilled steak or fish, or 2 eggs cooked any way.

Tropical Breakfast Smoothie   *(Stage 2)*

2 cups	Coconut milk (canned is acceptable but must be unsweetened); if it's too rich, dilute with
1 cup	water
1	Peach or 2 slices pineapple or 1 mango
6 to 9	Strawberries
3 tbsp	Synd-X Slimming Protein Powder or whey protein powder
1/3 cup	Ice

Trim fruit and place all ingredients in blender and process until silky smooth. Sprinkle with dried coconut and cinnamon or ground almonds or LSA to serve.

Serves 2

Handy Tips to Keep You on Track

Vegetables are ideally eaten with every meal, either fresh as a salad, and/or cooked, or as leftovers from the night before. The vegetables may be replaced with 1 to 2 pieces of raw fruit at breakfast or lunchtime.

Keep it as simple as possible for breakfast, as this is usually a very busy time of the day. If you have a salad left over from the previous evening then you may want to use that at breakfast with grilled meat or canned fish.

The salad will remain fresh overnight if you store it in an airtight container and it does not have dressing applied. Otherwise prepare strips, chunks or bite size pieces of salad (such as celery, snow peas, carrots, bell peppers, cauliflower and broccoli florets, bean sprouts, any type of lettuce, green beans, baby spinach leaves, watercress, spring onions or radish). Trim, wash and cut as desired and do enough to take for your lunch in an airtight plastic container.

Salad Recipes

Salads are very good for the liver and will promote weight loss. To help reduce hunger, we are combining as many of the food groups as possible in our salads to create a "First Class Protein Salad". Thus these salads can be considered a complete meal.

Any of the salads can be served with fresh cooked meat (or cold serves of this), poultry, cheese, eggs or seafood, but sometimes it is more convenient (especially for a workday lunch) to eat just a bowl of salad, and know that you are still eating a complete protein meal. We are also including salads that can be prepared well ahead of time, and that will stay fresh for several days, if stored in an airtight container without a dressing applied, in the fridge.

Planning ahead always makes meal times a lot easier and will help you to avoid being caught out with only take away foods around.

Salads will store in the fridge, for a few days prior to use.

Sun-Dried Tomatoes & Bean Salad   (Stage 2)

14oz (400g)	Beans, (cooked or canned), drained and rinsed
7oz (200g)	Sun-dried tomatoes, roughly chopped, drain off the oil
7oz (200g)	Black olives, deseeded and chopped
1 cup	Feta cheese, crumbled
1 tsp	Lemon rind, grated plus juice of ½ lemon
½ tsp	Cracked black pepper and sea salt
½ cup	Basil leaves, fresh and roughly chopped
1 - 2	Garlic cloves, crushed
½ cup	Pepitas (green pumpkin seeds), chopped
½ cup	Brazil nuts, or other nuts of choice, chopped
1 tbsp	Cold pressed olive oil

Preparation

Whisk together the oil, lemon juice, rind and pepper and salt and garlic.

Combine all of the other ingredients in another large bowl.

Pour on oil and lemon juice mixture and toss gently. This salad can be served on whole lettuce leaves as a complete meal, or as a side salad for fish and poultry.

Serves 4.

This bean salad will keep for several days in an airtight container in the fridge. Store the dressing in a jar in the fridge and do not apply dressing until you are ready to eat the stored salad.

This salad can be eaten on its own as a meal, as it contains 3 of the essential vegetarian food groups to provide a first class protein. It is an ideal salad to use as a workplace lunch.

Zesty Beetroot and Carrot Salad (Stage 1)

1 large	Raw beetroot, peeled and grated or sliced into small julienne pieces
2 large	Carrots, peeled and grated
1 large	Avocado, chopped
½ cup	White cheese (such as feta, ricotta or cottage), crumbled
1	Red onion, finely chopped
2 tbsp	Fresh mint and basil leaves, finely chopped
1 tsp	Lemon rind, grated
2 tbsp	Cold pressed olive oil
1/3 cup	Lemon juice
½ tsp	Chili flakes (optional)

Salt and pepper to taste

Preparation

Combine all ingredients.

This salad is ideal to serve with warm cooked lamb or beef, or as a side dish for grilled fish. It will store in the fridge for 2 days.

Serves 4 to 6.

Mixed Bean Salad   *(Stage 2)*

1	Three or four bean mix or any beans of your choice, canned or cooked
1	Lebanese cucumber, washed and diced
1	Red onion, sliced
1 large	Tomato, diced
1	Capsicum (bell pepper), de-seeded and cut into fine strips
2 sticks	Celery, leaves and all, chopped
1/3 cup	Fresh parsley, chopped
1/3 cup	Fresh basil, chopped
1 cup	Feta or mature cheese, chopped

Dressing

¼ cup	Balsamic vinegar, or apple cider vinegar
¼ cup	Cold pressed olive oil

Preparation

Drain and rinse the beans. Mix and combine the vegetables, herbs and cheese. Shake dressing ingredients together, and gently fold into the salad mixture.

This bean salad is a very filling protein meal served on its own with lettuce and carrot sticks. It will store in fridge for 2-3 days.

Serves 4

Tabbouleh Salad (Stage 3)

½ cup	Burghal (cracked wheat) or cooked brown rice if you are gluten intolerant
½ cup	Sunflower seeds
½ cup	Blanched almonds
1 tbsp	Sesame seeds
1 medium	Red onion, chopped
4 cups	Fresh parsley, chopped
4 cups	Fresh mint leaves, chopped
¼ cup	Fresh lemon juice
¼ cup	Cold pressed olive oil
3 medium	Tomatoes, chopped (Roma or vine-ripened tomatoes are best)

Preparation

Prepare the burghal by soaking in cold water for at least an hour. Drain well and remove as much moisture as possible using paper towels. This mixture should be as dry as possible.

Toss all ingredients together, except the lemon juice and oil, and refrigerate.

Place oil and lemon juice in a bottle or jar, season with salt and pepper to suit your own taste, shake well and toss through salad just prior to serving.

Serves 4 to 6.

This salad can be eaten on its own as a meal, as it contains three of the essential vegetarian food groups to provide a first class protein.

Rice Salad   (Stage 3)

4 cups	Brown rice, cooked, still warm, rinsed and drained
¼ cup	Sultanas
1	Green apple, chopped
½ cup	Spring onions, chopped
½ cup	Red capsicum (bell pepper), chopped and de-seeded
½ cup	Raw cashews or blanched almonds, chopped
½ cup	Sunflower seeds or hemp seeds
½ cup	Pepitas (green pumpkin seeds), chopped

Mix together all the above ingredients in a salad bowl

Dressing

½ cup	Cold pressed olive oil
1/3 cup	Apple cider vinegar
2 tbsp	Soy sauce
1 to 2 cloves	Garlic, crushed
2 tsp	Curry powder, commercially prepared, or your own recipe for curry powder, if preferred
½ teaspoon	Cracked black pepper and sea salt

Preparation

Mix dressing ingredients into a screw top jar and shake together.

Add the dressing mixture while the rice mixture is still warm. Store in the fridge in a sealed container. If you want it to last longer, store some separately from the dressing and keep the dressing in a jar until needed.

This rice salad will keep for several days in an airtight container in the fridge. It can be eaten on its own as a meal, as it contains 3 of the essential vegetarian food groups to provide a first class protein (a grain, a seed and a nut) *Serves 4 to 6.*

Salads that are best made just prior to serving

Spicy Salad with Cool Dressing (Stage 1)

1 cup	Red radishes, washed well and thinly sliced
½ cup	Coriander (cilantro), chopped
½ cup	Turnip, grated
1	Red or green capsicum (bell pepper), thinly sliced
1	Red onion, thinly sliced
1 cup	Celery, thinly sliced
1-2 small	Red chiliies, de-seeded and thinly sliced (optional)

Cucumber dressing

1	Lebanese cucumber, chopped
10oz (300ml)	Unsweetened plain or Greek yogurt
½ cup	Fresh mint leaves, chopped
1 tbsp	Fresh lemon juice
1 tbsp	Olive oil, cold pressed

Preparation

Process all of the dressing ingredients in a blender until smooth. Combine all salad ingredients in a bowl and drizzle dressing through the salad mixture until combined.

Taste tip: This cucumber dressing is also suitable to use as a side condiment for hot and spicy curries, and is delicious with Cajun dishes. Serve with a few cucumber and celery sticks and dip them in the dressing. This salad will be good for your liver and speed up your metabolic rate.

Serves 4 to 6

Spinach and Cheese Salad   (Stage 1)

4.5oz (125g)	Baby spinach leaves, with stems trimmed off
7oz (200g)	Parmesan, feta or mozzarella cheese, chopped
14oz (400g)	Chick peas, canned, rinsed and drained (optional)
1	Red capsicum (bell pepper), de-seeded and thinly sliced
1	Red onion, thinly sliced
½ cup	Basil leaves, chopped
¼ cup	Pepitas (green pumpkin seeds), chopped
½ cup	Raw nuts - hazelnuts, walnuts or macadamia, chopped

Dressing

¼ cup	Apple cider vinegar
2 tbsp	Cold pressed olive oil
1 tsp	Seeded mustard
1 clove	Garlic, crushed

Cracked black pepper and salt to taste.

Preparation

Place all salad ingredients in a bowl and toss together.

Place all dressing ingredients in a screw top jar and shake until well mixed. Pour dressing over salad just before serving.

Serves 4 to 6

Cabbage, Cucumber and Mint Salad (Stage 1)

14oz (400g)	Lebanese cucumber
1	Red onion, chopped
1 tsp	Coarse salt or sea salt
½ small	Cabbage, chopped finely (Chinese or Savoy ideal)
1	Carrot, grated
3 tbsp	Fresh mint leaves, chopped
1 tbsp	Sesame seeds toasted
½ cup	Walnuts, chopped
¾ cup	Natural cheese, of your choice, chopped (optional)

Dressing

1 tsp	Lemon rind, finely grated
2 tbsp	Cold pressed olive oil
½ cup	Fresh lemon juice
1 tsp	Nature Sweet Sugar Substitute or pinch stevia powder
1 tsp	Garlic, crushed or minced (optional)

Preparation

Mix salad ingredients together.

Place all dressing ingredients in a screw top jar, and shake until well mixed.

Pour dressing over salad ¼ hour before serving and refrigerate until ready to serve.

Serve with hard boiled eggs, fish or BBQ meats.

Serves 6

Liver Cleansing Salad (Stage 1)

1 cup	Broccoli florets
1 cup	Celery stalks and leaves - diced
1 cup	Red or green capsicum (Bell peppers) - diced
1 cup	Green beans - chopped
4 to 6	Spring onions - tops and all, chopped
½ cup	Snow peas - trimmed
1 cup	Parsley - chopped
1	Cucumber

A few red cherry tomatoes to garnish

Dressing

½ cup	Cold pressed sesame oil or olive oil
1 tbsp	Fresh garlic – crushed (optional)
½ cup	Freshly squeezed lemon juice
½ tsp	Dried cumin

Cracked black pepper and sea salt to taste

Put all ingredients into a jar, with the lid on shake until well mixed.

Preparation

Blanch broccoli in boiling water for 1 minute, drain, run under cold water and drain again.

Score cucumber skin with a fork and rinse under cold water and dice. Toss all ingredients together.

Serves 6 - 8

You can halve the ingredients for a small salad. This salad will last 1 to 2 days and even longer if you do not add the dressing to the stored salad. If you still have some left over, toss it in a pan with a little shredded cabbage for a stir-fry.

Nice and Spicy Salad   *(Stage 1)*

1 cup	Mung bean sprouts
1	Cucumber, thinly sliced
½ cup	Spring onions, chopped
1 medium	Red onion, thinly sliced
1 medium sliced	Capsicum (Bell pepper), de-seeded and thinly
¼ cup	Fresh coriander (Cilantro), chopped
7oz (200g)	Firm tofu, cubed and steamed prior to adding to salad, or else select equivalent amount cheese such as feta or mature cheese, chopped
2 small	Red chiliies, de-seeded and finely sliced (optional)
¾ cup	Raw Brazil nuts or cashews or almonds, well chopped
1 tbsp	Toasted sesame seeds

Dressing

1 tbsp	Hot chili sauce
2 tbsp	Soy sauce
1.5 cups	Cold pressed olive oil
2 cups	Sugar free tomato paste
2 tsp	Fish sauce
2 tsp	Nature Sweet Sugar Substitute or pinch stevia powder
¼ tsp	Ground ginger powder or fresh ginger, chopped

Preparation

Combine all salad ingredients. Combine all dressing ingredients in a screw top jar and shake, or place in blender and blend until mixed well, then drizzle over salad before serving

---

This salad dressing is also very tasty when added to some hot cooked noodles or pasta as a meal.

Serves 6

Very Low Carb High Protein Salad (Stage 1)

1 cup	Lettuce, torn
1 cup	Rocket, chopped
½ cup	Spinach leaves, chopped
½ cup	Cucumber, sliced
½ cup	Celery stalks and leaves, sliced
½ cup	Mushrooms, sliced
3 tbsp	Bean sprouts
1	Tomato, chopped
2	Radishes, chopped
2	Spring onions, sliced
7 oz (200g)	Parmesan or white cheese
4	Hard boiled eggs

Dressing

2 tbsp	Cold pressed olive oil
1 tbsp	Hummus

Juice of one lemon or lime

Pepper and sea salt to taste

Preparation

Mix all salad ingredients together and toss.

Mix all dressing ingredients together until well combined. Pour over the salad when ready to eat.

Serves 4 to 6

Spinach and Avocado Salad   *(Stage 1)*

2 cups	Raw spinach, chopped
1 – 2	Garlic cloves, chopped (optional)
4 tbsp	Spring onions, sliced
2	Hard-boiled eggs, quartered
1	Tomato, chopped
1 large	Avocado, cubed

Dressing

2 tsp	Fresh lemon or lime juice
2 tsp	Apple cider vinegar (good quality)
2 - 3 tbsp	Olive oil

Preparation

Shake dressing ingredients in a jar with tight lid.

Mix/toss salad ingredients in a bowl and drizzle over the dressing.

Serves 4 to 6

Chef's Salad   *(Stage 1)*

1 cup	Lettuce leaves, washed and torn
1 handful	Rocket leaves, chopped
½ cup	Canned chickpeas or beans
1	Red onion, chopped
½ cup	Button mushrooms, chopped
½	Red capsicum, chopped
½ cup	Celery stalks and leaves, chopped
1 cup	Fresh basil, chopped
1	Tomato, chopped
2oz	Cold lamb or chicken, diced or salmon or tuna
2	Hard boiled eggs, quartered

Preparation

Combine ingredients, and toss in dressing of choice.

Serves 4 to 6

Fruit and Nut Salad   *(Stage 2)*

1	Red apple, diced, skin on, core out
1	Green apple, diced, skin on, core out
1 cup	Celery stalks and leaves, diced
1 large	Avocado, diced
1	Red onion in thin half rings
7 oz (200g)	Fresh pineapple, chopped
1 cup	Parsley, chopped finely
½ cup	Fresh mint, chopped
1 cup	Fresh basil, chopped
1 cup	Pecans or walnuts, chopped

Dressing

3 tbsp	Olive oil
2 tsp	Apple cider vinegar
½ tsp	Mustard

Preparation

Mix all salad ingredients together.

Place dressing ingredients in a glass screw lid jar and shake to combine well. Pour dressing over the salad and serve.

Serves 6

Healthy and Slimming Lunches

Salmon and Avocado   (Stage 1)

7-8oz (210g)	Canned pink salmon
1	Avocado, chopped
1	Red onion, sliced
½	Cucumber, sliced
½ cup	Fresh basil leaves, chopped
½ cup	Fresh parsley, chopped
¼	Lettuce, chopped or equivalent amount of rocket leaves

Season with black pepper and sea salt and juice of half a fresh lemon

Don't discard bones from salmon, as they contain an easily absorbed form of calcium. Mash the bones into the fish. Can toss all ingredients together or arrange on plate.

Serves 2

Cold Roast Meat Salad Lunch   (Stage 1)

4oz (125g)	Cold roast meat left over from a roast dinner, sliced
1 medium	Carrot, grated
½ cup	Coriander, chopped
1 cup	Rocket leaves
1	Capsicum (Bell pepper), sliced
2	Celery stalks and leaves, sliced
1 cup	Fresh mint, chopped
1	Tomato, sliced
¼ cup	Almonds, chopped
Sea salt and fresh pepper to taste	

Preparation

Mix salad ingredients and drizzle with cold pressed olive oil and freshly squeezed lemon juice.

Serves 1 to 2

Hard Boiled Eggs   *(Stage 1)*

2	*Hard-boiled cold eggs, cut into quarters*
½ cup	*Coriander, chopped*
½	*Red onion, finely chopped*
1 cup	*Lettuce or Rocket, torn*
½	*Cucumber, sliced*
½	*Capsicum (Bell pepper), sliced*
½ cup	*Parmesan cheese, grated*
1	*Tomato, quartered*

Preparation

Serve with a handful of alfalfa or bean sprouts.

Drizzle over cold pressed olive oil and apple cider vinegar or lemon.

Serves 1

Tasty Chunky Tomato Lentil Soup   *(Stage 1)*

28oz (810g)	*Fresh tomatoes or canned chopped tomatoes*
1 cup	*Red lentils, soaked for one hour in 2 cups of boiling water*
1 cup	*Celery stalks with leaves, chopped*
2 tbsp	*Fresh basil leaves, chopped*
1 cup	*Coriander, chopped*
½	*Chili, chopped finely (optional)*
2 tsp	*Paprika*
½ cup	*Fresh parsley, chopped*

1 large	Onion, chopped
½ tsp	Cracked black pepper
½ tsp	Rock salt or sea salt
2 tbsp or more	Tomato paste
2-3 tsp	Cold pressed olive oil

Garlic, chopped according to your personal taste

Preparation

Brown the onion and garlic in a small amount of oil. Then add to all other ingredients in a large pan. Simmer gently until all is tender for approx. one hour.

Add more water if necessary. Season to taste before serving. This soup can be served chunky, or if preferred smooth - purée with a hand held food processor. Serve sprinkled with chopped parsley.

Suitable to freeze in meal size portions Serve tomato and lentil soup, with a tossed salad (sprinkle chopped nuts and sesame seeds through the tossed salad)

Serves 6.

Lamb Loin Chops with Salad   (Stage 1)

2 – 4	Chops, grilled
1 cup	Rocket leaves, chopped
1	Red onion, chopped
½ cup	Fresh mint leaves, chopped
½ cup	Mushrooms, chopped
½ small	Cucumber, sliced
1	Celery stalk and leaves, chopped
1	Tomato, sliced
1	Red capsicum (Bell pepper), sliced

Sea salt and fresh pepper to taste

Preparation

Toss salad ingredients together. Drizzle salad with fresh lemon juice or apple cider vinegar and cold pressed olive oil.

Serves 1 to 2.

Grilled Steak   (Stage 1)

Choose a piece of steak that is lean and fresh and grill according to taste.

Serve with a large tossed salad with a variety of raw vegetables.

Serves 1

Shellfish & Avocado with Spicy Dressing(Stage 1)

1 cup pieces	*Lettuce leaves, or rocket torn into bite size*
7-8oz (210g)	*Fresh or canned prawns, shrimp or crab meat, drained*
1	*Avocado, chopped*
1 small	*Lebanese cucumber, diced*
2 - 3	*Spring onions, chopped, or 1 red onion, chopped*
1	*Red capsicum (Bell pepper), chopped*
½ cup	*Celery stalks and leaves, chopped*
½ cup	*Fresh coriander, chopped*

Dressing

You can have a simple dressing of cold pressed olive oil and freshly squeezed lemon juice.

Alternatively choose the following spicy elaborate dressing consisting of -

½	Avocado
¼ cup	Sugar free mayonnaise or Homemade Creamy (See page 96 for recipe)
1 tsp	Seeded mustard
2-3 tsp	Cold pressed oil
2-3 tsp	Fresh lemon juice or apple cider vinegar
2-3 tsp	Tomato paste
1 tsp	Horseradish sauce
1 tsp flat	Nature Sweet Sugar Substitute or pinch stevia if you desire to sweeten the dressing
1 pinch	Chili flakes or one small fresh chili chopped finely (optional)

Preparation

Toss salad and seafood together. Blend dressing ingredients all together in a food processor then pour over the salad.

Store dressing in the fridge in a screw top jar for up to 4 days.

Serves 2.

Tomato & Basil Salad with Chili Dressing (Stage 1)

4	Roma (egg shaped) or vine-ripened tomatoes, cut into quarters
1	Red capsicum (red bell pepper), de-seeded and thinly sliced
1	Red onion, medium sized, thinly sliced
½ cup	Fresh coriander, chopped
2	Sticks of celery with leaves, sliced
¼ cup	Peanuts
¼ cup	Sesame seeds, dry roasted
8	Fresh basil leaves, chopped.

Toss all ingredients together.

Dressing

1 tbsp	Chili sauce, sweeten with a pinch of stevia or 1 tsp Nature Sweet Sugar Substitute if desired
2 tbsp	Soy sauce
2 tbsp	Cold pressed sesame seed oil or olive oil
1 tbsp	Tomato paste
2-3 cloves	Garlic crushed (optional)
2 tsp	Fish sauce
½ tsp	Cracked black pepper and sea salt

Preparation

Combine all ingredients in a screw top jar and shake well.

Pour over salad just before serving. Store remainder in fridge.

Serves 2 to 3

Sardine Dip with Fresh Vegetables (Stage 1)

1 can	Sardines in brine or spring water
1 clove	Garlic, crushed (optional)
10	Black olives, pitted
½ cup	Parsley, chopped
½ cup	Coriander, chopped
1 tbsp	Apple cider vinegar or fresh lemon or lime juice
1 tbsp	Cold pressed olive oil
	Black pepper to taste

Preparation

Place all ingredients in food processor until combined.

Serve with sticks/slices of fresh celery, capsicum, snow peas and carrot sticks.

Serves 1

Fish and Vegetable Combo   *(Stage 1)*

7-8oz (220g) Tuna, mackerel or salmon, can, drained

1 cup   Feta cheese, crumbled

1 clove   Garlic, crushed

1   Celery stalk with leaves, chopped

3 tbsp   Fresh parsley, chopped

3 tbsp   Fresh basil, chopped

1 tbsp   Cold pressed olive oil

½ cup each   Zucchini, broccoli, leeks and mushrooms, steamed

Pepper and salt to taste

Preparation

Mix all ingredients in a large serving dish and toss.

Serves 2

Tuna & Vegetable Sticks with Cucumber Dip (Stage 1)

4-5oz (125g) Tuna, mackerel or salmon in brine, canned, drained

1   Lebanese cucumber, grated

½ cup   Natural unsweetened full fat yogurt

1 handful   Rocket leaves

2 tbsp   Fresh mint, chopped

1-2 cloves   Garlic crushed, or

½   Red onion, chopped

2 tbsp   Fresh chives, chopped

Salt and pepper to your taste

Plenty of raw vegetable sticks, such as celery, carrot, cucumber or capsicums, (bell peppers) and snow peas.

Preparation

Combine cucumber with all the other ingredients and mix well.

Dip vegetable sticks into dip and enjoy. Refrigerate any leftovers for later.

Serves 1 to 2.

Boiled Egg, Avocado & Mustard Dressing (Stage 1)

2	*Hard boiled eggs, chopped*
½ cup	*Walnuts*
½ cup	*Bean sprouts or alfalfa sprouts, washed*
½ cup	*Coriander (cilantro), chopped*
½	*Red onion, chopped*
1	*Avocado, chopped*
2	*Celery stalks with leaves, chopped*

Dressing

1 tbsp	*Sugar Free Mayonnaise or Fresh Homemade Creamy Sugar Free Mayonnaise (see page 96)*
1 tbsp	*Seeded mustard*
2 tbsp	*Fresh orange or lemon juice*
1 tbsp	*Apple cider vinegar*

Preparation

Place all dressing ingredients in blender and process until smooth. Finally add 3 tbsp cold pressed olive oil, just letting it drizzle in while blender is still going.

Taste and add a little salt and black pepper if desired.

Dressing will keep in fridge in screw top jar for a few days.

To serve, pour dressing over chopped avocado and eggs with bean sprouts and celery sticks on the side. *Serves 2.*

Recipes

Uncooked Stuffed Tomatoes (Stage 1)

2 or more	Tomatoes, large - vine ripened are great
3-4oz (100g)	Crab meat or shrimps, cooked, (canned is OK if unable to get fresh), drain
¼ cup	Carrot, grated
2 tbsp	Fresh peas or fresh lightly steamed asparagus
6 or more	Black olives, pitted and finely chopped
1 tbsp	Coriander, (Cilantro), chopped
1 tbsp	Fresh basil leaves, chopped

Cut a small lid from tomatoes and gently scoop out flesh and seeds. Mix all other ingredients together and spoon into tomato shells.

Dressing

Flesh and seeds from tomatoes

¼ cup	Cold pressed olive oil
1 pinch	stevia powder or ½ tsp Nature Sweet Sugar Substitute
1 tbsp	Fresh dill, chopped
1–2	Garlic cloves, chopped (optional)

Pepper and salt to taste.

Preparation

Blend flesh and seeds from tomatoes and garlic clove until smooth, fold in other ingredients.

Pour dressing into stuffed tomatoes, and drizzle remainder over a generous serve of mixed green leaves or and any other green salad vegetables that you fancy.

Serves 2.

Paprika Chicken Drumsticks   (Stage 1)

8	Chicken drumsticks, free range or organic
1 tbsp	Wholegrain mustard
1 tsp	Garam masala
1 tsp	Chili flakes
1-2 tsp	Paprika
3 tbsp	Cold pressed olive oil

Salt and pepper to taste

Preparation

Combine all ingredients in a bowl and add drumsticks. Turn drumsticks until well oiled.

Chicken can be barbecued or grilled, or place in oven covered in foil for 45 minutes.

Remove foil for last 15 minutes.

Serve with strips of red and green capsicums (bell peppers), cooked broccoli and a large green salad.

These drumsticks freeze well, so double the recipe if you like.

Serves 4.

Cold Roast Meat with Salad   (Stage 1)

Slice desired amount of leftover cold roast meat. Place meat on a serving plate and serve with green leaf salad. The salad mixture should contain several varieties of lettuce, rocket, beetroot leaves, spinach and silver beet leaves, watercress and flat parsley leaves. Wash salad leaves, then spin or pat dry.

Dressing

This dressing will cover about 9oz (250g) of salad leaves

| ½ cup | Olive oil |
| ¼ cup | Apple cider vinegar |

¼ cup	Lemon juice
¼ cup	Flat leaf parsley, very finely chopped
2 tsp	Dijon mustard

Preparation

Shake together in a screw top jar and store in fridge.

Serves 4.

Salmon, Onion & Cucumber Salad   (Stage 1)

7-8oz (210g)	Salmon or tuna, canned, drained
4	Roma (egg-shaped) or vine-ripened tomatoes, quartered or sliced
1	Celery stalk with leaves, chopped
1 med	Red onion, finely sliced
2 med	Lebanese cucumbers, halved and cut into chunks
2 tbsp	Fresh coriander, chopped
2 tbsp	Fresh basil leaves, chopped
½ tsp	Black pepper and sea salt
½ tsp	Chili flakes
1 tsp	Balsamic vinegar
1 tbsp	Cold pressed olive oil

Preparation

In a flat salad bowl, layer the salad ingredients, sprinkling with seasoning as you layer them.

Drizzle oil and vinegar over top, gently shake bowl, cover and stand in fridge for at least half an hour.

Serve with salmon or tuna – eat enough to satisfy your hunger. This salad will store in fridge for 2 days.

Serves 1 to 2.

Boiled Egg and Snow Pea Salad   *(Stage 1)*

2 - 4	Hard boiled eggs, peeled and cooled

Salad

9oz (250g)	Green beans (or ½ green and ½ butter beans), washed
9oz (250g)	Snow peas, washed
1 med	Red onion, thinly sliced or chopped
¼ cup	Sunflower seeds
¼ cup	Pumpkin seeds, shelled
½ cup	Grated parmesan cheese

Salt and pepper to taste

Dressing

1-2 cloves	Garlic, crushed or minced
1 tbsp	French mustard
2 tbsp	Lemon juice, freshly squeezed
1/3 cup	Cold pressed oil
2 tbsp	Fresh parsley, chopped

Preparation

Cut beans and snow peas into 2inch (5cm) pieces. Blanch beans and snow peas in boiling water for 1 minute. Rinse immediately under cold water and drain.

Mix with all other salad ingredients.

Whisk all dressing ingredients together in a bowl, pour over salad and toss gently. Serve with eggs.

Serves 2.

Sliced Chicken Breast with Salad   (Stage 1)

1	Chicken breast grilled or roasted, sliced – served hot or cold

A good serve of a fresh garden salad or left over salad.

Serves 1.

Chicken and Vegetable Soup   (Stage 1)

4	Chicken drumsticks, remove skin and fat
2 cups	Carrot, chopped
2	Tomatoes, chopped
½ cup	Fresh parsley, chopped
½ cup	Fresh basil, chopped
1 cup	Parsnip, chopped finely
1 cup	Swede, chopped finely
1 cup	Turnip, chopped
1 cup	Celery, chopped finely
3	Garlic cloves, chopped finely
1 large	Onion, chopped

Preparation

Brown the onion and garlic cloves in 2 tsp olive oil in a pan

Place all ingredients in a large pan and barely cover with chicken or vegetable stock. Bring to boil and simmer for one hour until tender.

Remove chicken bones and leave meat in soup.

Season with black pepper and sea salt to taste.

Suitable to freeze in serving portions.

Serves 4

Grilled Fish with Peas & Pepper Salad (Stage 1)

1 fillet	Fresh fish of your choice per person - grilled

Salad

½ cup	Fresh or frozen peas
½ cup	Fresh mint leaves, chopped
1	Red capsicum (bell pepper), de-seeded and cut into strips
½ cup	Celery stalk and leaves, chopped
1 cup	Fresh parsley, chopped
1	Carrot sliced into sticks
½	Red onion, chopped
1 tbsp	Sesame seeds or hemp seeds

Season of black pepper and sea salt

Preparation

Simmer or steam peas and red pepper until just tender

Drain and toss with sesame or hemp seeds and dress with cold pressed olive oil and apple cider vinegar or fresh lemon juice.

Serve with celery and carrot.

Salad can be served either hot or cold.

Salad serves 2.

Lentil Patties with Vegetables   (Stage 1)

1 cup	Dried red lentils
2 cups	Water
1-2 tbsp	Curry powder, according to taste

A little cold pressed olive oil for cooking

1 whole	Egg lightly beaten
1 tbsp	Crunchy natural peanut butter, unsweetened
1 tbsp	Sesame seeds or hemp seeds

Extra hemp seeds for coating patties

Preparation

Rinse lentils under running water, then place in pan with new water, bring to the boil and simmer for about 15 minutes or until all water is absorbed.

Blend lentils and curry powder until smooth. Add peanut butter and seeds and mix well. Refrigerate mixture for about 30 minutes to firm up.

Shape into about 6 to 8 patties. Coat in extra hemp seeds.

Heat oil in a pan and cook patties about 5 minutes on each side or until nicely browned.

Serve patties with stir-fried vegetables, or a fresh green salad.

Freeze any leftover patties for a future meal.

Serves 3.

Weekend BBQ Lunch with Salads   (Stage 1)

Prepare ahead 3 to 4 salads from the salad selection in this book. Make enough for your family and guests. Prepare the salads that will keep in the fridge for a day or so, then you can have leftovers the next day.

For the barbecue allow per person –

1	Lentil patty (today you can call it a burger)
1 piece	Lean steak, thinly sliced and sprinkled with ground oregano and lemon juice
1	Chicken drumstick – or chicken kebab marinated in soy sauce

The meat can be prepared and refrigerated a couple of hours before guests arrive.

Chicken marinade

Slightly warm and mix together

⅔ cup	*Soy sauce, (sugar free)*
1 tsp	*Nature Sweet Natural Sugar Substitute or 2 pinches of stevia to taste*
1 tbsp	*Peanut butter, sugar free*
1 tbsp	*Sesame Oil*

Preparation

Coat the chicken and leave to stand for about 1 hour.

Drumsticks can be cooked in a pan in the oven until tender.

Kebabs go on the BBQ with the steak and burgers.

Serve meat with salads and finish off with a nice mixed fruit platter.

Coleslaw Salad (Stage 1)

This salad is simple to prepare and easy to take to work for lunch. It is nice and light served with a can of drained seafood or left over roast meat.

Toss all together.

¼	*Cabbage – Chinese or Savoy are best, shredded*
6	*Spring onions, chopped or finely sliced*
1	*Celery stalk and leaves, chopped*
1 small	*Red chili, de-seeded and finely chopped (optional)*
½ cup	*Fresh mint, coarsely chopped*
1 cup	*Fresh parsley, coarsely chopped*
¼ cup	*Coriander (cilantro), coarsely chopped*
1	*Carrot, grated*

Dressing

¼ cup	Fresh lemon juice
1 tbsp	Dijon mustard
½ cup	Cold pressed sesame or olive oil

Preparation

Toss all salad ingredients together.

Mix all dressing ingredients in a screw top jar and keep in refrigerator. Dressing can be added just before serving, or in the morning if more convenient, to take to work.

Serves 4 to 6.

Deviled Eggs with Olives & Sprouts (Stage 1)

2	Eggs, hard boiled
¼ cup	Sugar free mayonnaise, or Homemade Creamy Sugar free Mayonnaise (recipe on page 96)
1 tsp	Seeded mustard
1 tbsp	Fresh chives, chopped
¼ cup	Fresh coriander, finely chopped

A few drops of Tabasco sauce

Pinch of paprika

Black pepper and sea salt to taste

Preparation

Cut eggs in half lengthways and remove yolk.

Mash egg yolks then stir in all other ingredients.

Spoon the mixture back into the egg halves and serve with a mix of snow pea sprouts, onion sprouts and alfalfa sprouts and about 6 seeded black olives. — *Serves 1 to 2.*

BBQ Chicken Salad   (Stage 1)

2 cups	Assorted green leaves, chopped
½ cup	Coriander (cilantro), chopped
½	Red onion, chopped
1	Tomato, sliced
½	Cucumber, sliced
1	Celery stalk with leaves, chopped
1 small	Avocado, diced
½ cup	Mung bean sprouts, washed

Chunks of barbecued chicken

Preparation

Combine all ingredients and dress with olive oil, apple cider vinegar or lemon juice — *Serves 2*

Tuna or Salmon Salad   (Stage 1)

7-8oz (210g)	Tuna or salmon in brine, drained
1 cup	Lettuce or assorted green leaves, chopped
½ cup	Celery with leaves, chopped
½ cup	Coriander (cilantro), chopped
1	Tomato, sliced
¼	Cucumber, sliced
2	Spring onions, sliced, or ½ red onion, chopped
1	Hardboiled egg, quartered

Preparation

Combine all ingredients and add a dressing of cold pressed olive and apple cider vinegar, or lemon juice. If you do not feel like fish you can replace it with feta or ricotta cheese or another natural cheese of your choice.

Serves 2.

Bean Salad   (Stage 2)

1	14oz (410g) Three bean mix, canned, or any canned legumes of your choice. (I like to buy organic beans and soak them in water overnight to make my own)
1	Red onion, thinly sliced
1	Capsicum (Bell pepper), seeded and thinly sliced
1/3 cup	Bean sprouts
½ cup	Fresh mint and basil leaves, chopped
½ cup	Pepita seeds (pumpkin seeds), chopped or hemp seeds
½ cup	Pine nuts or chopped almonds

A good squeeze of lemon juice

Pepper and sea salt to taste

Preparation

Gently mix all ingredients together. Serve with lettuce. Add feta or mozzarella cheese as a garnish.

Drizzle over some cold pressed olive if desired.

Make enough for 2-3 serves as this will keep refrigerated in an airtight container for 2 days.

Sardine Spread for Crackers or Bread (Stage 2)

1 can	Sardines in brine or spring water
1 clove	Garlic, crushed (optional)
10	Black olives, pitted
½ cup	Parsley, chopped
½ cup	Coriander (cilantro), chopped
1 tbsp	Apple cider vinegar or fresh lemon juice
1 tbsp	Cold pressed olive oil

Black pepper to taste

Preparation

Place all ingredients in food processor until combined. Spread onto 2 or 3 Ryvita crackers, gluten free crackers or 1 slice of bread. Serve with celery and carrot sticks.

Serves 1.

Canned Fish with Tabouli Salad   (Stage 2)

2 tins	Sardines, herrings or kippers – in brine – mash the bones, do not discard them

Salad

3 med	Tomatoes, de-seeded and chopped
1/3 cup	Sunflower seeds
5 tbsp	Burghul, soaked in water for half an hour, drain and pat dry
1 large	Red onion, chopped finely
1	Celery stalk with leaves, chopped
4 cups	Fresh parsley leaves, chopped
2 cups	Fresh mint leaves, chopped

Salt and pepper to taste

Dressing

¼ cup	Fresh lemon juice
¼ cup	Cold pressed olive oil

Preparation

While the burghul is soaking, prepare all other ingredients and then toss all ingredients together until well mixed. Store covered in fridge.

Tabouli will keep for 2-3 days. Serve with dressing. *(Salad serves 6)*

Prawns and Mango Salad   *(Stage 1)*

6 large	Prawns (shrimp), cooked and peeled
1 cup	Mixed green leaves
1	Tomato, cut into bite size pieces
1 small	Lebanese cucumber, thinly sliced
½	Small red onion, sliced
½ cup	Fresh mint, chopped
1	Mango, sliced
1 cup	Fresh coriander, chopped

Handful bean sprouts to garnish

Dressing

½ cup	Fresh Homemade Creamy Sugar free

Mayonnaise (see page 96 for recipe)

1 tbsp	Tomato paste, sugar free
½ tsp	Tabasco sauce
½ tsp	Horseradish sauce
3 pinch	Ground oregano

Preparation

Mix dressing ingredients in blender, until well combined.

Store left over dressing in screw top jar or bottle in fridge.

Place all salad ingredients on serving plate.

Top with prepared prawns and drizzle with dressing.

Serves 2 to 3.

Frittata with Lettuce Cups of Salad (Stage 1)

3 large	Whole eggs, lightly beaten
2 cups	Mixed vegetables of your choice, chopped and cooked until almost tender, such as sweet potato, cauliflower, broccoli, corn, spring onions, chives, mushrooms, green beans, peas, carrot and zucchini
2 tbsp	Fresh parsley, chopped
2 tbsp	Fresh basil, chopped
2 tbsp	Sugar free mayonnaise or Homemade Creamy Sugar Free Mayonnaise (See page 96 for recipe)
1 cup	Parmesan cheese, grated

Ground black pepper and sea salt to taste

Preparation

Pour 2 tsp cold pressed olive oil into a fry pan. Mix all ingredients together and pour into pan, except parmesan cheese. Sprinkle the parmesan cheese over the top of the mixture.

Cook over medium heat gently until mixture is set – usually 5-7 minutes, depending on thickness of mixture. Mixture should be brown on bottom, excessive heat will burn bottom before mixture is set.

Now place pan under hot grill, just long enough to brown top.

Let stand in pan for a few minutes to settle and firm up. Slice and serve warm, with lettuce cups containing any leftover salad, or a mixture of grated carrot and beetroot and sliced tomato.

Serves 3.

Tasty Bean and Olive Salad   *(Stage 2)*

14oz (400g)	Cannelloni beans (canned or cooked), washed and drained
3 to 4	Vine-ripened tomatoes, chopped
3-4oz (100g)	Black de-seeded olives, roughly chopped
¼ cup	Pepitas (green pumpkin seeds), chopped
2	Celery stalks with leaves, chopped
¼ cup	Pine or pistachio nuts or other nuts of choice
½ cup	Parmesan cheese
1	Red onion, chopped
2 tbsp	Hemp seeds or sesame seeds

Sprinkle of pepper and sea salt

2 tbsp	Fresh basil leaves, roughly chopped
1 cup	Fresh rocket leaves, chopped
1 clove	Garlic, crushed (optional)
¼ cup	Lemon juice, freshly squeezed
1 tbsp	Lemon rind, finely grated

A drizzle of cold pressed olive oil

½ cup	Parmesan cheese, to garnish

Preparation

Brush tomatoes with cold pressed olive oil and bake uncovered in a moderate to hot oven for about 30 minutes taking care not to burn. Cool and chop roughly.

Place all ingredients into a bowl and toss to gently combine.

A large serve is a meal on its own.

Garnish with ½ cup parmesan cheese.

Leftovers can be stored in a sealed container in the fridge and used as a salad with meat or fish.

Serves 4 to 6.

Vegetable and Bean Soup   (Stage 2)

1 large	Red onion, chopped
1 to 2	Cloves garlic, crushed (optional)
1	Bay leaf
14oz (400g)	Red kidney beans, canned and drained
½ cup	Pearl barley (avoid if gluten intolerant and replace with ½ cup corn kernels)
1	Fresh chili, chopped
14oz (400g)	Pumpkin, peeled and chopped
4 medium	Zucchinis, sliced
1 large	Carrot, sliced
14oz (400g)	Tomatoes, canned, or 4 fresh tomatoes
2	Celery stalks with leaves, chopped
1 tbsp	Toasted sesame seeds

A drizzle of cold pressed olive oil

Preparation

Heat oil in pan and brown onion and garlic until soft.

Place all ingredients into large pan and barely cover with water – about 35oz (1 litre) or vegetable stock.

Bring slowly to boil then simmer gently with lid on for 30 minutes, or until all vegetables are tender.

If preferred you may blend or process this soup until smooth.

Sprinkle with chopped parsley and toasted sesame seeds to serve.

Freeze any leftovers.

Serves 6 to 8.

Vegetarian Burger (Stage 2)

½ cup	Soybeans (canned or cooked) or tofu
1	Carrot, grated
½ cup	Fresh basil, chopped
1	Whole egg
½ cup	Peanuts or cashews, chopped
½ cup	Toasted sesame seeds
1	Onion, finely chopped or grated
1	Celery stalk with leaves, chopped
2	Garlic cloves, crushed
1 tsp	Dill seed

Sea salt and pepper to taste

Preparation

Mix all ingredients with beaten egg.

Add ½ tsp salt and cracked black pepper and dill seed. Shape into patties. Warm olive oil in pan and brown patties on both sides, or bake until dry and brown. Serve with fresh salad.

Serves 1 to 2

Jacket Potatoes with Filling (Stage 3)

| 2 large | Potatoes, boiled or baked in jacket until tender |

Filling

7-8oz (210g)	Beans or lentils, canned
1 med	Onion, thinly sliced
1 tbsp	Fresh coriander, chopped
½ cup	Chives, chopped
½	Capsicum, (bell pepper), de-seeded and finely chopped
Pinch	Chili powder (optional)
2 tsp	Black pepper and sea salt

Preparation

Put all ingredients, except potatoes, into a saucepan, mix and gently heat through.

Cut a cross in top of each potato and squeeze to open. Spoon bean mixture into and over potatoes. You can replace the beans with cooked lean beef or lamb mince if desired.

Potatoes can be topped with grated parmesan cheese if desired. Serve with a generous serve of coleslaw salad.

Serves 2

Easy In-A-Rush Lunch   (Stage 3)

2 slices	Sour dough, wholegrain or gluten free bread or 3 crackers
2	Vine-ripened tomatoes
2	Spring onions, chopped finely
1 tbsp	Cold pressed olive oil

Pepper and sea salt

Preparation

Toast bread and then drizzle olive oil or hummus over the toasted bread.

Layer bread with slices of freshly cut tomato and spring onion. Sprinkle with pepper and salt

Eat this with one can of sardines, smoked oysters or crab meat.

Serves 1 to 2.

Vegetable and Seafood Stir-Fry   (Stage 1)

25oz (700g)	Uncooked king prawns or mixed seafood of your choice (fish pieces, calamari, octopus, mussels etc.)
1 -2 tbsp	Cold pressed olive oil
1	Onion, cut into wedges
7oz (200g)	Broccoli, cut into small pieces
2	Garlic cloves, crushed (optional)
1	Fresh chili or 1 tsp chili flakes
1	Red capsicum (bell pepper), sliced
5oz (150g)	Small mushrooms or tomatoes, chopped
2 tsp	Fresh ginger, grated
1 ½ cups	Stock – vegetable, chicken or fish stock
2 tbsp	Fresh squeezed lime juice
1 ½ tbsp	Chili sauce (optional)
1 tbsp	Fish sauce

Preparation

Peel and de-vein prawns and wash all seafood.

Heat 2 tsp oil in pan or wok.

Add seafood and stir-fry over high heat for 1 minute, or until browned, then remove.

Heat remaining oil, add capsicum (bell pepper), tomato, onion, fresh chili or chili flakes and broccoli, stir-fry for 2 minutes.

Add mushrooms, garlic and ginger, stir-fry for 1 minute Add seafood and remaining ingredients, stir-fry for 2 minutes, or until tender.

Serve with fresh green salad. — Serves 4

Accompaniments to Meals

Linseed, Sunflower Seeds & Almonds (LSA)

Much has been written about the tremendous health benefits of linseed (flaxseed) and indeed many types of seeds, such as sesame seeds, chia seeds, pumpkin seeds and hemp seeds in our diets. Since the introduction of "LSA" - Linseed, Sunflower seeds and Almonds some time ago, many of us have added this mixture to our favorite recipes such as smoothie drinks, cereals, soups, dips, casseroles, biscuits and desserts, and in fact anything which can include a meal substance. LSA is an excellent source of healthy essential fatty acids, minerals, fibre and vitamin E. Many types of seeds have anti-cancer properties and are low in carbohydrate.

LSA Recipe   (Stage 1)

3 cups	Linseeds (flaxseeds)
2 cups	Sunflower seeds
1 cup	Almonds

(For smaller quantities use tablespoons instead of cups)

Preparation

Use a coffee grinder or food processor, and grind to a fine meal. Store in an airtight container in the refrigerator or freezer. It will last forever in the freezer. Use as required but re-seal to retain freshness.

LSA can be sprinkled over your usual cereal or on toasted bread with tahini or nut paste.

If you enjoy fresh fruit for breakfast, chop up a banana, some melon, pears, apples, oranges, kiwi fruit, strawberries, or any of your preferred fruits, and sprinkle with LSA.

Gomasio Recipe   (Stage 1)

Gomasio is a Japanese condiment made from sesame seeds and salt. It is extremely high in calcium and other beneficial minerals. Gomasio adds a delicious flavor to any savory meal. Try it instead of salt!

1 part	Sea salt
23 parts	Hulled sesame seeds

Preparation

Heat a heavy frying pan. Add sea salt and stir gently as it dries out. Add sesame seeds, combine with the salt. Stir continuously until the sesame seeds are golden brown; be careful not to burn them. The seeds are ready when they can be crushed easily between your thumb and finger. Pour the mix into a grinding bowl. Grind the mixture, keeping it quite coarse, as it is nice to chew. Allow to cool before storing in airtight container

A delicious variation of Gomasio is -

2 tbsp	Dry roasted sesame seeds, crushed
2 tbsp	Water
2 tbsp	Tamari sauce

This is great with steamed vegetables, or over half an avocado filled with seafood.

Sea Vegetable Condiment   (Stage 1)

1 oz (30g)	Dry arame
1 tbsp	Vinegar
½ tbsp	Shoyu sauce
3 drops	Chili oil or ½ tsp chili flakes
½ tbsp	Sesame oil
½ bunch	Fresh chives, chopped into ¼ inch (½ cm) lengths

Preparation

Soak the arame in boiling water for 5 minutes. Drain well and set aside. Mix the vinegar, shoyu and chili.

Heat a frying pan, add the sesame oil. Sauté the chives for 1 minute. Add the arame and cook for another 2 minutes. Pour in the liquids. Simmer gently until most of the liquid has gone. Spoon into a small bowl and serve with your vegetables or grains.

Serves 6

Tahini Dressing *(Stage 1)*

4tbsp	Tahini
2 cloves	Garlic, crushed
1 tbsp	Lemon juice
1tbsp	Tamari
1 tbsp	Cold pressed olive oil

Add cold water to thin out the dressing

Preparation

Place all ingredients in a jar and mix well and shake, or mix in a blender. The tahini will make the dressing quite thick, so add cold water to make to your desired consistency.

Tofu Dressing *(Stage 1)*

7oz (200g)	Fresh silken tofu, drained
2 tbsp	Lemon juice
2 tbsp	Cold pressed olive oil
1 tbsp	Tamari
1 tsp	Miso
4 tbsp	Tahini

Add water to liquefy

Makes 1 cup

Preparation

Blend all ingredients until smooth. Serve on any hot vegetables, or as a salad dressing.

Olive Tapenade (Stage 1)

5.3oz (150g)	Green or black pitted olives
4	Anchovies (rinsed)
2	Garlic cloves, peeled
2 tbsp	Capers
1 tbsp	Lemon juice

Freshly ground black pepper

Cold pressed olive oil

Preparation

Place all ingredients in a blender. Dribble olive oil into the mix while blending until smooth consistency

Homemade Creamy Sugar-Free Mayonnaise (Stage 1)

2 large	Egg yolks
2 tsp	Vinegar (organic apple cider)
2 tsp	Fresh squeezed lemon juice
½ tsp	Mustard powder
¾ cup	Cold pressed virgin olive oil
1 pinch	Paprika or for an extra bite, cayenne pepper

Pinch of sea salt

If you want it to taste slightly sweet use 2 pinches stevia or ½ tsp Nature Sweet Sugar Substitute

Preparation

Place all ingredients, except the oil, in a blender and blend until well combined.

Then when the blender is still operating, add half the oil, drop by drop, until the mixture becomes a creamy consistency. The rest of the oil can be added more quickly in a fine stream now.

Should the mixture begin to curdle, add 1 tsp of either very hot or icy cold water, and this should make it revert back to a creamy consistency.

Natural Mayonnaises   (Stage 1)

Mayonnaise Version One

Great with seafood cocktails and salads such as coleslaw.

½ cup	Sugar free mayonnaise
¼ cup	Apple cider vinegar or lemon juice
2 tsp	Tomato paste
½ tsp	Horseradish sauce
1 tsp	Garlic, minced (optional)
¼ tsp	Black pepper and salt
Pinch	Chili powder or 2 to 3 drops Tabasco sauce

Shake all together in a screw top jar and refrigerate

Mayonnaise Version Two

½ cup	Sugar free mayonnaise
¼ cup	Apple cider vinegar or lemon juice
1 tsp	Dry mustard powder
1 tsp	Nature Sweet Natural Sugar Substitute or 2 pinches of stevia to taste
½ tsp	Ground oregano
½ tsp	Black pepper and salt

Shake all together in a screw top jar and refrigerate

Stocks

The best vegetables for stock are carrots, leeks, onions (with skin), parsley stalks, celery (not the leaves), garlic, celeriac, and sweet corn. To add a delicious full body flavor to your stocks, try roasting the vegetables first in the oven, then place them in the saucepan and continue as per recipe.

Wash all your produce to ensure it is free from bacteria and dirt. With chicken stock, remove all the offal and wash thoroughly with cold running water. Fish stock only needs to be cooked for approximately 20 minutes, as it can become gluey. All the stocks in this book make approximately 8-9pints (5 liters) of stock

Vegetable Stock *(Stage 1)*

2 medium	Onions, cut in half (do not peel)
2 large	Carrots, chopped into 3 pieces
½ head	Celery (leaves removed)
0.8inch (2cm)	Fresh ginger, sliced
2.5 inch (6cm)	Kombu seaweed stick (optional)
2 cloves	Garlic
1	Bay leaf
7	Black pepper corns
1 tsp	Sea salt
2 tbsp	Cold pressed olive oil
24 cups	Water

Preparation

Place oil into large saucepan on high heat, do not burn the oil. Place all other ingredients (except water) into the pan. Stir until the smell of the vegetables releases. Add the water and bring to the boil, then simmer gently for 1 hour. Strain the liquid. Toss away the solids and keep what you need. Pour into containers when cool and freeze.

Fish Stock   (Stage 1)

Make sure your fish smells pleasant and don't use oily fish
(such as sardines, mackerel or any smoked fish)

4	Prawn heads or 1 large fish head
1 tsp	Sea salt
1	Red chili, chopped
1 bunch	Coriander (cilantro)
1 bunch	Parsley
2 large	Onions
5	Peppercorns
4	Garlic cloves
2.5 inch (6cm)	Kombu seaweed stick (optional)
24 cups	Water

Preparation

Place all ingredients in a large saucepan and bring to the
boil. Skim off any scum. Return to a gentle simmer for 20
minutes. Strain and throw away all the solids. Allow to cool
and remove any fat that comes to the surface. Freeze the
remainder (some in small containers), as it is great to cook
rice/grains etc.

Chicken Stock   (Stage 1)

1	Free-range chicken, or chicken pieces
2 medium	Onions, cut in quarters (leave skin on)
1	Chili, chopped
2 medium	Carrots, cut in half
½	Celeriac root, peeled and halved, or ½ head of celery, leaves removed and halved
2 cloves	Garlic
1	Bay leaf

1 bunch	Parsley
1 cup	Fresh basil
1 pinch	Rock salt
2 tbsp	Cold pressed olive oil
1 tsp	Freshly ground black pepper (optional)
24 cups	Water

Note: Offal can make your stock bitter

Preparation

Wash meat thoroughly if you are using uncooked chicken. Place oil into large saucepan, on high heat, do not burn. Place all ingredients (except water and parsley) into the pan. Stir until the smell of the vegetables releases (about 5 minutes). Add the water and the parsley. Bring to the boil (not vigorously), then simmer gently for approx 2 hours. Remove solids and allow to cool. Remove fat from surface (free-range chicken fat is more like jelly). Freeze remainder of stock within two days.

The Family Roast

Roast meat can be "liver friendly" if you follow the guidelines below. Roasted meats are a very good source of protein for those with Syndrome X. All of the roasts can be used as main courses for dinner and the leftovers used as cold lunch meats. This is much healthier than using preserved delicatessen meats such as ham, devon, sausage, corn beef, smoked salmon or turkey, or fritz.

Use tender cuts of meat trimmed of excess fat such as

- Scotch Fillet
- Eyepiece of Silverside (not corned)
- Eyepiece of Pork or Beef is an ideal cut
- Leg of Lamb
- Baby Veal, legs or fillet
- Chicken or Turkey

Roast Beef   (Stage 1)

55-70oz (2kg) Beef
2-3 tsp   Grainy mustard
2-3 tsp   Horseradish sauce
2-3 tsp   Soy sauce

Preparation

Mix all the ingredients to form a paste, and rub all over the meat before placing the meat in the oven.

Cook at 200°C/390°F (no higher), until the meat is cooked to your personal taste.

When the meat is cooked, remove it from the oven and retain the meat juices for gravy.

Leave the meat to stand or rest before carving. Cover the meat whilst it is standing/resting to retain heat.

Using meat juices makes a rich gravy of your choice to pour over carved meat.

If you like garlic you can make several tiny cuts in your beef and push in slivers of fresh garlic before rubbing on spicy paste.

Serve with baked vegetables and salad.

Roast Lamb   (Stage 1)

Rub the lamb over with olive oil and sprinkle on a mixture of herbs such as rosemary and mint leaves. Cook the lamb as directed for beef.

Serve with sugar free mint sauce and baked vegetables and salad.

Roast Pork   (Stage 1)

55-70oz (2kg) Scotch fillet of pork
2   Green apples - peeled, cored and cooked in a
             little water with 2 whole cloves.

Preparation

When apples are cooked, remove the cloves and drain off all liquid.

Add to the apple pulp 1-teaspoon grainy mustard and ½ teaspoon dried oregano.

Spread this mixture over the pork and place meat in an oven and cook as directed for beef.

Serve sliced with gravy made from juices of the meat and your preferred gravy mixture.

Roast Veal (Stage 1)

Leg of baby veal or 55-70oz (2kg) fillet of veal

Brush meat sparingly with soy sauce, oregano and thyme. Make small slits in the meat and add sprigs of mint or basil into the slits. Add cloves of garlic if desired. You can stud the meat with a few whole cloves.

Place the meat in the oven.

Sauce

3.5oz (100g) Button mushrooms, sliced very thinly

2 Spring onions, finely chopped

Preparation

Cook mushrooms and onions in the residual juices from the pan then thicken with a little plain flour to make a nice pouring sauce.

Season to taste before pouring over the sliced roasted veal – delicious!

Roast Poultry (Stage 1)

Buy free range or organic poultry of your choice (if preferred boned and prepared). Rub a few extra mixed herbs on the outside of the meat, and either section the bird or place it whole in the oven with olive oil. Place 2 cloves of garlic and half a lemon inside the chicken cavity. Squeeze ¼ of lemon on the chicken. Cook until meat is tender.

Serve with light gravy made with meat juices (take fat off) and the flavor of your choice.

Serves 4 to 6

Rack of Lamb with Lemon and Rosemary (Stage 1)

2	Racks of Lamb (12 chops in total)
3	Garlic cloves
6 sprigs	Rosemary
6 sprigs	Fresh mint
2 tbsp	Cold pressed olive oil

Juice of 1 fresh lemon

Black pepper to taste

Fresh mint and rosemary to garnish

Preparation

Preheat oven to 400°F (200°C).

Peel and halve garlic.

Cut a tunnel between the meat and the bone and fill with garlic, lemon juice and some rosemary.

Pierce the lamb and insert rosemary and mint over the lamb's surface.

Place racks in a baking dish, sprinkle with pepper and olive oil.

Bake for 40 minutes or until cooked through.

Cut rack into cutlets.

Serve with steamed green vegetables and a salad.

Serves 4 to 5

Wilted Greens (Accompaniment)   (Stage 1)

This is a great accompaniment to any meat dish.

1 bunch	*English spinach, washed, larger stems removed*
2 bunches	*Baby bok choy, washed, quartered length ways*
1 bunch	*Asian broccoli, washed and cut into finger size lengths*
1 tsp	*Lemon skin / zest (finely grated)*
3 tbsp	*Tamari*
1 tbsp	*Toasted sesame seed oil or cold pressed olive oil*

Preparation

Place all greens into a saucepan with fresh water and the lemon zest.

Heat saucepan until steaming.

The water from the washed greens will be enough to steam/stir-fry greens.

Warm sesame oil and tamari.

Remove vegetables from the heat when they are wilted, bright green and slightly crisp.

Place greens on a serving dish.

Pour warmed tamari and oil over greens.

Serves 2 – 6 (6 if served with another dish)

Healthy and Slimming Dinners

Coriander and Lemon Chicken   *(Stage 1)*

2 large bunches	Coriander, chop leaves coarsely
2	Garlic cloves, finely chopped
2" (5cm)	Ginger, thinly sliced
2	Lemons, juiced
½ tsp	Garam masala
1 tsp	Paprika
½ tsp	Chili powder (optional)
1 tsp	Cumin seeds
1 tsp	Sea salt
35oz (1 kg)	Chicken thigh fillets
2 tbsp	Olive or coconut oil
5	Fresh tomatoes, chopped

Preparation

Combine coriander, garlic, ginger, lemon juice, garam masala, paprika, chili, cumin and salt, and mix well

Add chicken, toss well and leave in marinade for 30 minutes, stirring from time to time

Heat oil in pan, add chicken with marinade and cook over moderate heat until tender

Add tomatoes and cook for 10 minutes over low heat. Serve with steamed vegetables and salad.

Serves 4 to 6

Stir-Fry Chicken and Vegetables *(Stage 1)*

2	Chicken breasts (or 2 thighs per person), cut into strips
1 stalk	Fresh lemon grass, remove outside layers to the soft core, and chop finely
1 tsp	Black peppercorns, coarsely ground
2 small	Chiliies, de-seeded and finely chopped (optional)
1" (2.5cm)	Fresh ginger, peeled and finely chopped
2	Lime leaves, finely chopped
2	Limes juiced
4 tbsp	Tamari sauce
2 tbsp	Hemp seeds
2 cups	Broccoli, chopped into bite sized pieces
1 ½ cups	Green beans, washed
2 cups	Carrot, cut into thin strips
1	Onion cut into eights
1 cup	Small mushrooms, rinsed and halved
4	Fresh coriander roots, washed and finely chopped
1 large	Garlic clove, finely chopped (optional)
2 tbsp	Cold pressed olive or flaxseed oil
1 tbsp	Sesame oil

Preparation

Heat oil in wok or large fry pan.

Add chicken, stir until cooked and remove from pan.

Add chiliies, ginger, coriander root, garlic, lemon grass, peppercorns and lime leaves to the pan and stir.

Add the vegetables and lime juice and tamari, stir until almost cooked. Add chicken and stir until blended through the vegetables. *Serves 2*

Chicken Satay (Stage 1)

12	Chicken thigh fillets
2 tbsp	Chili sauce (can use less if desired)
1 tbsp	Coconut oil or ghee
1	Garlic clove, crushed
2 tbsp	Fresh coriander, chopped

Peanut Sauce

9oz (250ml) Chicken stock

½ cup (4.5oz) Natural unsweetened crunchy peanut butter

1 tsp   Sesame oil

¼ cup   Chili sauce – if you want sweet chili sauce add ½ tsp of Nature Sweet Natural Sugar Substitute or 2 pinches stevia

1 tbsp   Lemon juice

Combine all ingredients in a pan, simmer and stir until sauce is slightly thickened.

Preparation of Chicken

Cut chicken fillets into 4 strips lengthways.

Combine chicken with other ingredients in a bowl and refrigerate for 3 hours, or overnight.

Thread chicken strips onto skewers.

Grill or BBQ until chicken is brown and tender.

Serve with peanut sauce and a fresh green salad and steamed baby bok choy.

Serves 6

Indian (Goan style) Chicken Curry (Stage 1)

1" (2.5cm)	Fresh ginger, peeled and grated
¼ whole	Nutmeg, grated finely
¼ cup	Shredded coconut
4	Cloves
1	Cinnamon stick
1 tsp	Ground coriander
1 tsp	Ground turmeric
½ tsp	Cardamom seeds, crushed
½ tsp	Whole black peppercorns
5 cloves	Garlic, finely chopped
2 small	Red chiliies, finely chopped (optional)
¾ cup	Water or chicken stock
1 large	Onion, finely chopped
8	Skin-less chicken drumsticks
1 tsp	Sea salt
2 tbsp	LSA (Linseeds, sunflower seeds and almonds)

Preparation

Toast coconut in a large, non-stick fry pan, over high heat, stirring constantly for about a minute.

Add ground nutmeg, cloves, cinnamon, coriander, turmeric, cardamom and peppercorns – stirring constantly for approx 2 minutes.

Place mixture into a blender, blend until finely ground.

Transfer mixture into a bowl.

Heat 1 tsp of the oil in a fry pan.

Add garlic, ginger and chiliies – cook for 2 minutes.

Place remaining oil in frypan, heat gently, add onion and cook until golden brown.

Stir in the chili mixture and LSA Add chicken, salt, spice mixture to the pan.

Cook over a medium heat for 5 minutes, stirring the chicken, to cover it with the spices.

Add remaining water or chicken stock and bring to the boil.

Reduce heat, cover and simmer until the juice of the chicken runs clear – about 30 minutes.

Turn the chicken frequently during cooking.

Delicious served on a bed of steamed spinach (about half a bunch per person).

Serves 4

Marinated Indian Lamb Cutlets   (Stage 1)

16	Lamb cutlets
1 tbsp	Fresh ginger, grated
2 tsp	Ground cumin
1 tsp	Fresh coriander, chopped, or ground coriander
1 tsp	Ground turmeric
½ tsp	Garam masala
1 tbsp	Lime juice
½ cup	Natural full fat yogurt
3 tbsp	Tandoori paste

Preparation

Trim excess fat from cutlets. Mix other ingredients in a shallow non-metallic dish. Add cutlets and coat meat with mixture.

Cover dish with plastic wrap and refrigerate overnight. Remove cutlets from the marinade. Brush grill with oil.

Cook cutlets over medium to high heat for 5 minutes each side, or to your liking. Serve with a large green salad. Serves 8

Lamb with Mint and Eggplant   (Stage 1)

1 medium	Eggplant, washed and cut into bite sized chunks
2 tbsp	Cold pressed olive oil
17-18oz (500g)	Lean lamb fillets, thinly sliced
2	Garlic cloves, chopped
2	Red chiliies, de-seeded and chopped
2 tbsp	Fish sauce
1 tbsp	Tamari
1/3 cup	Water
30	Fresh mint leaves
1 large	Onion, cut into thin wedges

Preparation

Place eggplant in a colander and sprinkle with salt, leave to drain for 20 minutes, rinse under cold water and drain well.

Heat oil in a large pan or wok.

Add lamb, onion, chiliies, and garlic, cook until browned.

Add eggplant and continue to cook for 5 minutes.

Stir in fish sauce, tamari, water and mint leaves and heat until eggplant is softened.

Serve with fresh green salad or wilted greens (see page 104 for recipe)

Serves 4

Quick Pork Casserole   (Stage 1)

1 medium	Eggplant, cut into one inch slices
2 tbsp	Olive oil
32oz (900g)	Pork fillets, cut into one inch cubes
1 large	Onion, chopped
2	Garlic cloves, crushed
1 large	Red and green capsicum (bell pepper) cut into one inch slices
28oz (810g)	Canned peeled tomatoes (no added sugar)
1 tsp	Dried oregano
1 tsp	Dried thyme
2 tsp	Dried basil
1	Bay leaf

Salt and pepper to taste

Preparation

Place eggplant on a board, sprinkle with salt, and leave for 20 minutes, rinse and pat dry

Heat oil in a large pan, cook pork quickly in small batches over medium to high heat until browned.

Drain on paper towels. Add onion and garlic to pan, cook for 2 minutes.

Add capsicums (bell peppers), cook for 4 minutes, stirring.

Return pork to pan with other ingredients. Bring to boil. Simmer for about 30 minutes, stirring occasionally

Serve with a large green salad.

Serves 6

Fish with Basil and Black Olives   (Stage 1)

1 tbsp	Olive oil
4	White fish fillets (ensure free of bones)
26oz (750g)	Spinach, washed, trimmed and chopped
1 tbsp	Lemon juice
½ tsp	Chili flakes or fresh chopped chili (optional)
1/3 cup	Cold pressed olive oil
1 clove	Garlic, crushed (optional)
2oz (60g)	Kalamata or similar olives
¼ cup	Basil leaves, shredded

Preparation

Heat oil in large fry pan, add fish and brown on both sides until just cooked.

Remove fish and keep warm.

Steam spinach until just tender.

Combine lemon juice, chili, extra oil, garlic, olives and basil in same pan, cook until hot.

Serve spinach topped with the fish and drizzle with oil mixture.

Serve with green salad.

Serves 4.

Poached Salmon Steaks with Herbs (Stage 1)

1 cup	Vegetable, chicken or fish stock
½ cup	Water
½ tsp	Dill, chopped
¼ tsp	Dill seed
1	Bay leaf
2	Salmon steaks
	Fresh dill and lemon slices for garnish
	Salt and pepper to taste

Preparation

Combine broth, water, bay leaf, chopped dill and dill seed in a large saucepan.

Add salmon and heat, then simmer for 4 to 5 minutes or until fish flakes easily with a fork.

Place salmon on plates, garnish with fresh dill and lemon slices.

Serve with mixed garden salad and dressing of cold pressed olive or flaxseed oil, and fresh lemon juice.

Serves 2

Cajun Fish   (Stage 1)

18oz (500g)	Thick fish fillets – John Dory, snapper, deep sea bream, mullet, swordfish or gem fish are all suitable
¼ cup	Cold pressed olive oil
2	Shallots or 1 small onion, finely chopped
2 cloves	Garlic, minced
1 tsp	Sea salt
½ tsp	Garam masala
½ tsp	Paprika
½ tsp	Cayenne pepper
½ tsp	Freshly ground black pepper
2 tbsp	Fresh parsley, chopped for garnishing

Preparation

Cut fish fillets into 2 inch cubes.

Mix oil, onion and all seasonings together in a bowl.

Add fish pieces and stir to thoroughly coat all pieces. Let stand for at least 15 mins.

Smear some extra olive oil in a pan and heat the pan.

Add fish in a single layer and turn often until fish is cooked.

Do not over cook fish.

Repeat with the remaining fish.

Drain fish on a paper towel. Serve hot with a cool green salad.

A squeeze of lemon juice is often a piquant addition just as you serve.

My son often adds a little plain yogurt and lemon or lime juice to the pan juices after cooking the fish, to make a very nice spicy, creamy, piquant sauce.

Note: Cajun seasoning is available ready prepared at many supermarkets. If you prefer to use these blends, sprinkle liberally over fish before cooking in oil. Be cautious with Cajun seasonings. Hot for some can be very hot for others. Remember you can always add more seasoning if desired.

Chicken, lamb and pork are delicious prepared Cajun style.

Moroccan Fish   (Stage 1)

2 tbsp	Cold pressed olive oil
1	Onion, chopped
3 cloves	Garlic, crushed
½ medium	Fennel bulb, washed and thinly sliced
¼ tsp	Fennel seeds
1 tsp	Garam masala
1 tsp	Ground cumin
17-18oz (500g)	Ripe tomatoes, washed and chopped
2 tsp	Tomato paste
4	Blue eye cod steaks or haddock/swordfish fillets
1 bunch	Fresh parsley, washed & chopped
1	Lemon, rind grated then juiced
Salt and pepper to taste	

Preparation

Heat 1tbsp oil in frying pan.

Add onion, garlic, cumin, garam masala, fennel and fennel seeds, stir-fry 2 to 3 minutes..

Stir in tomatoes, and cook for 2 minutes.

Add tomato paste, simmer for 15 minutes, stir occasionally, and set aside.

Heat remaining oil in fry pan.

Add fish and sear - brown quickly on both sides.

Transfer fish to kitchen paper and wipe out pan to remove excess oil.

Turn off the heat.

Lay most of the parsley on the bottom of the pan.

Place the fish in a single layer on top of the parsley. Sprinkle lemon rind and juice and season with pepper and salt.

Pour over the tomato sauce. Apply heat to simmer for 10 minutes.

Serve with steamed green vegetables (asparagus, spinach, beans etc) and garnish with parsley.

Serve a green salad on the side.

Serves 4

Spiced Prawns   (Stage 1)

17-18oz (500g)	Uncooked medium-sized king prawns
1 tsp	Turmeric
1 tsp	Ground cumin
1 tsp	Chili flakes
2 cloves	Garlic, crushed
1 tbsp	Lemon juice
1 tbsp	Cold pressed olive oil

Preparation

Shell and de-vein prawns, rinse prawn meat.

Combine all other ingredients, add prawns, and stir.

Refrigerate for one hour.

BBQ or grill prawns for 2 minutes each side.

Serve with steamed green vegetables and fresh salad.

Serves 2

Garlic Baked Cod, Green Beans & Tomatoes   (Stage 1)

4	*Good size pieces of blue eyed cod fillets*
9oz (250g)	*Green beans washed, topped & tailed*
1	*Onion, thinly sliced*
6	*Garlic cloves, thinly sliced (can use less if desired)*
4 tbsp	*Parsley, washed and chopped*
2 tbsp	*Olive oil*
14oz (400g)	*Tomatoes, chopped, with juice (may use canned)*
1 tsp	*Fresh or dried oregano*
1 cup	*Fresh basil, chopped*
15	*Black olives*
Plenty of freshly ground black pepper	
A little water	

Preparation

Mix beans, onion, garlic, pepper and olive oil together in a roasting pan.

Lay pieces of cod on top of the above mixture.

Spread tomatoes over the top of the fish.

Sprinkle with oregano and a bit more black pepper.

Place in a preheated oven (190°C/375°F) for 45 mins or until cooked.

Remove 2 to 3 times to use juice to baste the fish.

Add cold water if it begins to dry out too much.

Toss in the black olives and basil for the last 20 minutes of cooking time

Serves 4

Tempeh Burgers *(Stage 1)*

4 tbsp	Cold pressed olive oil
2	Onions, finely chopped
3 cloves	Garlic, finely diced
1-2	Red chilies, de-seeded and finely chopped (optional) 1tsp ground cumin
1 tsp	Ground coriander
4 cups	Tempeh, chopped finely or blended
2 tbsp	Fresh parsley, chopped finely
2	Eggs

Salt and pepper to taste

Preparation

Heat 2 tbsp oil in a fry pan Stir-fry onions until slightly golden, add garlic, chili, spices and cook for another minute Stir in tempeh and pepper and salt to taste .

Cook for another 2 minutes.

Remove all the cooked ingredients to a bowl and leave to cool.

Mix in parsley and the eggs, mix well.

Form into 4-6 patties.

Shallow-fry in the remaining oil in a non-stick pan, 4-6 minutes each side.

Serve as a traditional burger with salad and vegetables.

Serves 4-6

Low Fat Apricot Chicken   *(Stage 2)*

4 large	*Skin-less chicken fillets - trimmed of all fat*
2 tbsp	*Dried apricots, chopped*
2 tbsp	*Hazelnuts, chopped*
1 tsp	*Dried oregano*
1 tbsp	*Olive oil*

Preparation

Mix apricots, nuts and oregano.

Cut the chicken fillets to open out as flat as possible.

Lay one fillet out and sprinkle 1/3 of filling over the flesh.

Repeat with each fillet until you have a stack of 4 fillets.

Sprinkle top fillet with ground black pepper and a little extra dried oregano.

Tie fillets into a parcel shape with string and place carefully onto a greased oven dish.

Add 2 tablespoons of water or stock and bake in the oven, as directed, in preparing for roasting.

Bake about 1 hour or until tender.

When cooking is complete, retain the juices to pour over the meat as a gravy later on.

Slice your chicken parcel carefully with a sharp knife and enjoy your delicious seasoned chicken topped with the tasty meat gravy.

Serve with steamed green vegetables and fresh salad.

Note: If you can get free range organic chicken this is more delicious.

Serves 4.

Creamy Chicken Curry   (Stage 2)

Chicken mixture is best-made one day ahead. Add yogurt mixture before serving.

35oz (1 kg)	Chicken thigh fillets, fat trimmed
2 tsp	Ground cumin
¼ cup	Cold pressed olive oil
1 large	Onion, chopped
½ tsp	Garam masala
2 tsp	Curry powder (or preferred strength)
½ tsp	Ground cumin (or extra)
1 tsp	Ginger, grated
1 tsp	Nature Sweet Natural Sugar Substitute or 2 pinches of stevia
3-4oz	Natural yogurt
2 cups	Chicken stock
½ cup	Coconut cream (unsweetened)
1 tbsp	Lemon juice

Preparation

Combine all spices in a bag. Cut chicken into pieces and place in bag and shake well.

Heat oil in large pan and brown chicken all over.

Remove chicken from pan.

Add onions to pan and lightly brown. While stirring add spices, garlic, ginger and Nature Sweet/Stevia. Cook for about 1 minute.

Return chicken to pan, cover, reduce heat and simmer for 45 minutes or until chicken is tender, stirring occasionally.

Yogurt Mixture

Combine yogurt, coconut cream and lemon juice and add to chicken, reheat but do not boil. Serve with a Nice Cool Salad. *Serves 6*

Lemon Chicken Hotpot   (Stage 2)

35oz (1 kg)	Chicken thighs or breast fillets (remove skin)
1 tsp	Cracked black pepper and sea salt
1 tsp	Curry powder
3 tsp	Coriander - freshly chopped

Mix spices in a plastic bag, add chicken pieces and shake well.

Heat 1 tablespoon of cold pressed oil in a pan and brown chicken. Then place chicken in a casserole.

Now blend together:

1 ½ tbsp	Corn flour or potato starch
½ cup	Chicken stock
2 tbsp	Hemp seeds
¼ cup	Fresh lemon juice
2-3 tsp	Hot chili sauce with ½ tsp of Nature Sweet Sugar Substitute or 1 pinch of stevia
1 tsp	Soy sauce
2 tsp	LSA

Preparation

Stir this mixture over heat until it thickens a little - then add 2 teaspoons LSA and pour over chicken pieces.

Cover and cook at 390°F/200°C for about one hour or until chicken is tender.

Serve with steamed broccoli and sliced carrots and a green salad.

Serves 4 - 5.

Roast Pigeon or Quail   (Stage 2)

Buy clean and freshly dressed birds and wipe inside with paper towels.

Marinade for 4 - 6 birds

½ cup	*Balsamic vinegar*
¼ cup	*Cold pressed olive oil*
¼ cup	*Port or red wine*
2-3 tsp	*Soy sauce*
1 tsp	*Mixed dried herbs*

Preparation

Mix all ingredients together and pour over birds.

Cover and leave for at least an hour turning the birds occasionally.

Place birds in the oven and pour remaining marinade in the pan.

Bake at 180°C/355°F for 45 minutes - test with skewer and cook for another 15 minutes if required.

Meanwhile, lightly brown one chopped onion in a little oil, then add meat juices to pan and simmer until slightly thickened. Pour over birds and serve.

Serve with roast vegetables and fresh salad. — *Serves 4 - 6.*

Beef in Black Bean Sauce   (Stage 2)

26oz (750g)	*Lean rump steak – cut into strips*
1 tbsp	*Dry sherry*
2 tbsp	*Soy sauce*
2 tbsp	*Black bean sauce*
1/3 cup	*Cold pressed olive oil*
4	*Spring onions, sliced*
2	*Celery stalks, sliced*

1	Red capsicum (bell pepper), seeded and sliced
½ cup	Bamboo shoots, sliced
1 tsp	Curry powder

Preparation

Marinate beef strips in sherry, soy and black bean sauce, stir in flour and let stand for 30 minutes.

Heat oil in wok, add onions, bell pepper, celery, bamboo shoots and curry powder and sauté for 2 minutes.

Remove vegetables from wok with slotted spoon. Add meat to the remaining oil in wok and cook until browned and tender – approx 5 minutes.

Return vegetables to wok and heat through and serve with steamed carrot, broccoli and cauliflower.

Serves 4 – 6.

Green prawns can be used in place of steak for a change.

Lamb and Root Vegetable Soup   *(Stage 2)*

1	Shoulder of lamb, trimmed of fat
1 ½ liters	Water or vegetable stock
½ cup	Fresh rosemary, chopped
1	Carrot, sliced
1	Parsnip, diced
1	Turnip, sliced
1	Swede
2	Celery stalks and leaves, chopped
4 tbsp	Fresh parsley, chopped
1 cup	Fresh basil leaves
2	Garlic cloves, finely chopped (optional)

Salt and pepper to taste

Preparation

Place lamb in a large pot and add stock to cover. Season and bring to boil and simmer for 30 minutes, skimming the top to remove the fat.

Add swede, parsnip, carrot, turnip, herbs and celery. Simmer for 1 ½ hours.

Remove from heat, cool and refrigerate overnight.

Remove any fat from the surface.

Detach meat from the bones, cut into small pieces and return to soup.

Reheat and stir in parsley, garlic, salt and pepper and serve.

Serves 6.

Tuna Bake *(Stage 2)*

14-15oz (410g)	Tuna or salmon in brine, drained and broken into chunks
4	Hard boiled eggs, roughly chopped
1 cup	Vegetable or Chicken stock
½ cup	Soy mayonnaise or Homemade creamy sugar free mayonnaise (see page 96 for recipe)
1 tsp	Curry powder – commercial or your own recipe
¼ tsp	Black pepper & rock salt
2 tbsp	Spring onions, chopped
2 cups	Mashed sweet potato
1 tbsp	Cold pressed olive oil

Preparation

Mix mayonnaise, salt & pepper, curry powder and chicken stock together in a bowl.

In a casserole dish, layer the tuna/salmon, eggs, parsley and onions.

Pour the mixture over the layers then gently spread the mashed sweet potato over the top.

Brush the sweet potato with a little oil, roughen the top with a fork, and bake in a moderate oven for 30 – 40 mins until heated through and the topping is a golden brown.

Serve with plenty of cooked green vegetables or a green salad of your choice.

Serves 3.

Another option is to replace the tuna or salmon with an equivalent amount of canned crab meat or shrimps.

Cooking Meat

Any meat, poultry or fish, trimmed of all fat, will give you a complete protein meal. You can cook all of these meats by any method you choose, except for deep-frying.

If using a pan, use a healthy ceramic pan or a stainless steel variety and just oil with a little cold pressed olive oil. All types of seasonings can be added to the meats to enhance flavor. Here are some examples.

Lamb Chops, Fillets or Cutlets

Sprinkle with ground oregano, fresh mint leaves and a squeeze of lemon and leave to stand for ½ hour before cooking.

Spread lightly with tomato paste and sprinkle with a mixture of dried crushed basil, chopped fresh rosemary and ground black pepper.

Drizzle with a little cold pressed olive oil and sprinkle lightly with chili powder or sweet chili sauce (or even better, a hot chili sauce with a pinch of Nature Sweet Natural Sugar Substitute). Sprinkle with dried rosemary and lemon juice.

Beef Steaks and Fillets

Marinate for ½ hour in a mixture of ½ tsp of Stevia or Nature Sweet Natural Sugar Substitute, soy sauce and a dollop of natural peanut butter.

Press with cracked black pepper.

Spread with grainy mustard.

Marinate for ½ hour with a mixture of equal quantities of non-sweetened plum sauce, Worchester sauce, and chili sauce.

Sprinkle with Italian or Cajun spices and a squeeze of lemon juice.

Spread with minced garlic and horseradish.

Pork steaks, chops, fillets and spare ribs

Spread with a mixture of grainy mustard and apple sauce.

Spread with a mixture of soy sauce, honey and cracked black pepper.

Marinate for ½ hour in unsweetened plum sauce with a pinch of curry powder.

Chicken Fillets, Drumsticks and Wings

Marinate in soy sauce with some Nature Sweet Natural Sugar Substitute and sesame seeds added.

Sprinkle with lemon pepper and dried parsley, which are then rubbed and pressed into the meat. Sprinkle with mixed herbs, which are then rubbed and pressed into the meat.

There are many prepared marinades and spice mixtures that can be used, but try to choose those free of added sugar.

If you prefer, just trim the meat of all fat and cook it how you choose with no additives.

Serve with some of your salad of choice and top with your favorite salad dressing.

Casserole Cooking

Casserole cooking is easy and convenient.

Brown some onions in a little cold pressed olive oil.

Brown the meat of your choice before putting it into a casserole dish with as many vegetables as you choose.

Add a can of tomatoes or stock, cover and cook in a moderate oven until the meat is tender.

If you roll the meat in LSA before browning, it will help thicken the juices.

You can also drain a can of soy, kidney or cannelloni beans and add them to the casserole.

Casseroles freeze very well, so always make enough for a couple of meals to save you time in the future.

Soybean Dishes

Soybeans - served in any way (as cooked beans, tempeh or tofu) with rice and seeds or nuts, make a good source of first class of protein. Tempeh and tofu both have quite a mild flavor. Tempeh will take on any flavor you cook it with, so it makes a great additive to any dish.

Tempeh can be used as a meat substitute for most dishes that use meat. It can also be blended or liquidized and used in sauces, dips and dressings.

When made at home, tempeh can be made from different varieties of nuts and beans.

Rice Dishes

Rice is easy to digest and is free of gluten. Its nutritional value is greater when unpolished (brown). There are many varieties of rice: long and short grain, sticky, glutinous, brown, white, red, black and wild. Washing your rice until the water is clear makes it fluffy and helps to stop big clumps forming.

If using the reduction method of cooking in a saucepan or a rice cooker, always separate the grains before serving with a fork.

A rice cooker can be a fantastic addition to any household. They can be obtained from most large department stores and Asian grocery stores. Rice cookers can be used to make delicious one pot meals (no washing up).

Try using a homemade vegetable or chicken stock to cook your rice instead of water. It's fantastic!

Keep your portions of rice small as rice is high in carbohydrates, which is the thing to be minimized in those with insulin resistance.

Lemongrass and Tofu   *(Stage 1)*

This is great for BBQ's or on the grill

13-14oz (375g)	Firm tofu, cut into 24 cubes
2	Garlic cloves, peeled & crushed
1 knob	Fresh ginger, grated
2 tbsp	Soy sauce or tamari
2 tbsp	Cold pressed olive or sesame oil
1 stick	Lemongrass, cut off roots (peel the first 2 layers off) and chop finely
½ tbsp	Sesame seeds
1	Red capsicum (bell pepper), de-seeded & cut into 8 cubes
2 medium	Zucchini, wash and trim ends
2 medium	Japanese eggplants, wash and trim ends
8	Dry lemongrass stalks (to be used as skewers) or use regular skewers
½ cup	Sesame seeds, toasted
½ cup	Pine nuts or peanuts, toasted or raw
	Freshly ground black pepper

Preparation

Toss tofu, garlic, ginger, soy sauce, oil and chopped lemongrass.

Set aside to marinate.

Slice the zucchinis into halves, then cut each piece into four.

Repeat for the eggplant, make the slices smaller so you have 24 pieces altogether.

Sprinkle the eggplant pieces with salt and leave to stand for 30 minutes.

Drain the juices from the eggplant and pat dry with paper towel.

Cut roots off lemongrass, peel off the hard outer leaves.

Skewer one piece of bell peppers, zucchini and tofu, three of eggplant, one of tofu, zucchini and one more tofu.

Repeat with the remaining skewers (if the lemongrass is too flexible to pierce the firm vegetables, use a regular skewer).

Drizzle remaining marinade over the top and season with salt and pepper.

BBQ or char grill until golden brown for about 20 minutes.

Serve with toasted sesame seeds and nuts and a green leafy salad.

Makes 8 large skewers.

Tofu and Lotus Root Stir-Fry *(Stage 1)*

8	*Dried shiitake mushrooms, soaked in warm water for 30 minutes*
2 tbsp	*Cold pressed olive oil*
14oz (400g)	*Firm tofu, cut into bite sized pieces*
1 medium	*Onion, finely sliced*
1/3" slices	*Frozen/fresh lotus root*
1 small	*Head broccoli, washed and cut into florets*
3.5oz (100g)	*Snow peas, washed and trimmed*
1 tbsp	*Toasted sesame oil*
2 tbsp	*Toasted sesame seeds and pine nuts or peanuts*
Soy sauce to taste	

Preparation

Remove mushrooms from water, take off stems.

Heat olive oil and sesame oil in a wok or fry pan, add tofu and brown on both sides.

Remove tofu from pan and set aside.

Stir-fry onion, lotus root, broccoli, snow peas and mushrooms.

Fold through tofu when vegetables are tender but still crisp.

Serve with sesame seeds and toasted pine nuts and soy sauce.

Side salad of fresh greens.

Serves 3 to 4

Asian Stir-Fry Tempeh & Vegetables (Stage 1)

1 tbsp	Toasted sesame seed oil
1 tbsp	Sunflower seeds
1 tbsp	Sesame seeds
3 tbsp	Cold pressed olive oil or ghee
1 inch knob	Fresh ginger, grated
1 large	Onion, halved and roughly sliced
1	Red chili, de-seeded and thinly sliced (optional)
½ head	Broccoli, washed and cut into florets
1 cup	Fresh or frozen peas
6 pieces	Lotus root, halved
1 cup	Fresh corn cut from 1 corn cob
2 handfuls	Fresh green beans, washed, topped and tailed
4 tbsp	Tamari or light soy
2 cups	Vegetable or chicken stock
13oz (375g)	Tempeh, halved length ways then thinly sliced
1 bunch	Fresh coriander
1 cup	Pumpkin, thinly sliced

Preparation

Heat olive oil in a wok or large fry pan.

Toss in ginger, chili and onion, stir-fry for 3 minutes.

Add tempeh and cook until golden brown, stirring fairly constantly. Add a splash of stock if you need to.

Toss in half of coriander and all the vegetables.

Pour in stock and tamari.

Continue to cook on a high heat until vegetables are cooked, with a little bit of crunch.

Pour toasted sesame seed oil over vegetables and stir through.

Turn off heat.

Serve in big deep bowls.

Garnish with remaining coriander, sunflower and sesame seeds. *Serves 4 - 6*

Vietnamese Noodle Soup with Seafood (Stage 2)

1 small	Squid, cleaned and cut into bite size pieces
10-11oz (300g)	Firm fish fillet
7oz (200g)	Green prawns, shelled and de-veined
3.5oz (100g)	Scallops
2 tbsp	Cold pressed olive oil
6 small	Young Chinese broccoli stems, cut into 2 inches lengths, peel away any tough skin
1" (2.5cm)	Fresh ginger, peeled and grated
70oz (2 ltr)	Chicken stock
10-11oz (300g)	Fresh egg noodles
3	Spring onions, finely chopped
2	Lemons, cut into quarters
6 tsp	Soy sauce or tamari (maybe more depending on taste)
Fresh chili sliced (optional)	

Preparation

Heat stock in a large saucepan and leave on stove to simmer.

Bring another large saucepan of water to the boil and add egg noodles.

Cook for 2 minutes until tender, drain, keep cooking liquid.

Divide noodles between 6 serving bowls.

Return the noodle water to the boil, add broccoli and cook for 2 minutes.

Remove Chinese broccoli with a slotted spoon, discard water.

Add grated ginger to chicken stock for extra flavor.

Use a small strainer to put the seafood in and dip it into the simmering chicken stock, a bit at a time, hold in the stock until cooked, about 30-60 sec.

Distribute cooked seafood evenly among the bowls.

Bring chicken stock back to the boil.

Sprinkle spring onions evenly between the bowls.

Pour in hot chicken stock.

Serve chili, lemons and tamari as side dishes to be added as desired.

Serve with large garden salad.

Serves 6

Squid with Vegetables and Herbs (Stage 3)

2 tbsp	Cold pressed olive oil
2	Onions chopped
3	Garlic cloves, crushed
1	Fresh red chili, de-seeded and thinly sliced (optional)
2	Anchovy fillets

10oz (300g) Eggplant (aubergine), cut into 2.5cm cubes

4   Mint leaves, torn

5 tbsp   Fresh parsley, chopped (2 tbsp for garnish)

2   Zucchini, smallish, sliced

4   Ripe fresh tomatoes, quartered

3.5oz (100g) Roasted capsicum (bell peppers), roughly chopped

35oz (1kg) Squid, prepared and cut into small squares

Enough cooked rice for each plate

Salt and pepper to taste

Preparation

Heat 1tbsp of the oil in a large fry pan.

Add onion, garlic, chili and cook until softened.

Stir in anchovies, mash them so they can dissolve.

Add eggplant and cook for 5 minutes.

Toss in the mint, parsley and zucchini, allow zucchini to wilt.

Add tomatoes and capsicums (bell peppers), stir occasionally until vegetables are tender.

Heat remaining oil in another pan.

Just before serving toss in the squid, stir-fry on high heat, for about 90 seconds.

Remove squid with slotted spoon.

Place cooked rice on plates, add the vegetables, then the squid

Garnish with thinly sliced lemon, or parsley.

Serves 6

Spiced Rice (Stage 3)

2 tbsp	Cold pressed olive oil
1	Onion, peeled and diced
2 cups	Basmati rice, cleaned washed and drained well
1	Cinnamon stick
½ tsp	Sea salt
1 tsp	Cumin seeds
1 cup	Fresh green peas
4 tbsp	Sunflower seeds (dry roasted)
4 tbsp	Crushed almonds
3 cups	Stock

Preparation

Heat a heavy pan with a tight fitting lid and add the oil Sauté the onions, cinnamon, almonds and cumin until golden brown

Pour in the rice and stir gently to coat the rice in the oil for about 5 minutes

Bring the stock to a simmer in a separate saucepan

Add the simmering stock to the rice and cover with the lid

Turn the heat to very low and cook for 20 minutes

Take off heat altogether

Add the peas, replace the lid immediately – leave for 5minutes

Remove the lid and allow to stand for another 5 minutes

Fluff the rice with a metal fork (stops clumping)

Sprinkle with the dry roasted sunflower seeds

Serve as a side dish to meat, or is delicious on its own

Serves 5

Congee   (Stage 3)

2 handfuls	Short grain rice
4 cups	Chicken or vegetable stock
8 thin slices	Fresh ginger, 4 slices to be cut into slivers for serving with the meal
3	Spring onions, finely chopped
¼ tsp	Toasted sesame oil per serving
1 tsp	Sea salt
4 cups	Chicken or fish, cut into thin strips

Preparation

Wash the rice until the water runs clear.

Mix together the stock, salt and half the ginger in a large saucepan.

Add rice, mix well and bring to the boil.

Reduce to a simmer as low as possible (you can use a heat diffuser).

Cook for about 30 minutes.

While rice is cooking

Add ¼ inch of chicken stock to fry pan, bring to simmer.

Add strips of chicken or fish.

Cover with lid and simmer for 2 minutes, or until tender Stir chicken/fish into rice.

Serve in deep bowls topped with the remaining ginger, spring onions and toasted sesame oil.

Serves 6

Tempeh Curry (Stage 3)

9oz (250g)	Raw tempeh
2 large	Onions, cut into wedges
1 bunch	Fresh coriander (wash plant, separate root from leaves, keep leaves for garnish)
21oz (600g)	Pumpkin, cut into medium wedges, remove skin if desired
¼ cup	Sesame seeds, toasted
1 tsp	Toasted sesame oil
2 tsp	Red or green curry paste
2 tbsp	Tamarind paste (adds a tang)
14oz (400ml)	Coconut milk, unsweetened (canned)
14oz (400ml)	Vegetable stock
2 tbsp	Cold pressed olive or coconut oil
2	Lemons - cut each lemon into 3 pieces

Cooked rice for 6 persons

Preparation

Heat the oil in a wok or pan.

Stir-fry the tempeh until golden brown and set aside.

Add 1 tbsp new oil. Sauté the onions until brown

Add the washed & chopped coriander root, cook for 5 minutes

Add pumpkin and stir into the mixture

Stir the tempeh in gently

Add tamarind paste, coconut milk and stock and bring to a simmer

Cook uncovered until the pumpkin is tender and simmer to reduce the liquid

Serve on brown rice, garnish with lemon wedges and coriander leaves and sprinkle with sesame seeds - *Serves 6*

Chickpeas and Rice   (Stage 3)

The fresh chickpeas give this dish a delicious crunch.

14oz (400g)	Cooked chickpeas, drained and rinsed
14oz (400g)	Cooked rice
2-3tbsp	Cold pressed olive oil
2 large	Garlic cloves, peeled and crushed
2 tbsp	Dry roasted sunflower seeds
1	Red onion, finely chopped
1 inch	Fresh ginger, grated
1 ½	Lemon skins, (zested or finely grated), then juice the fruit from the lemons
1 bunch	Coriander, washed and chopped
7oz (200g)	Fresh or frozen peas
1 tsp	Garam masala
1 pinch	Dried chili flakes (optional)
2 tsp	Ground cumin
1 tsp	Sweet paprika

Preparation

Heat 2 tbsp of the oil in a large frying pan.

Add onion, garlic and grated ginger and cook for 5 minutes.

Add chickpeas, chili flakes and lemon rind and stir for about 30 seconds.

Add lemon juice.

Mix in the rice and fresh peas and stir for 1 minute and allow to cook until nearly all the juice is gone.

Add coriander, cumin, paprika and garam masala.

Serve in a warmed bowl with a large green salad Serves 4

Couscous and Vegetable Casserole (Stage 3)

¼ cup	Cold pressed olive oil
2	Brown onions, peeled and thinly sliced
4	Garlic cloves, peeled and crushed
1-2	Birds eye chiliies whole (optional)
3 tbsp	Tomato paste
35oz (1 ltr)	Vegetable stock or water
½ bunch	Coriander, washed and chopped
½ bunch	Parsley, washed and chopped
3 large	Tomatoes, quartered
1	Lemon, the skin finely grated, then juiced
5 tbsp	Sunflower seeds and pine nuts, dry roasted ground spices
1 tsp	Cumin
1 tsp	All spice
1 tsp	Turmeric
1 tsp	Sweet paprika
1 tsp	Black pepper
½ tsp	Ginger

1 serve of cooked couscous per person

2 cups hard vegetables such as celery, carrot, fennel, swede, turnip, parsnip etc., chopped bite size pieces

2 cups of soft vegetables such as eggplant, squash, green beans, zucchini, peas etc., chopped into bite size pieces

Preparation

Heat oil in large pot and add onions, chili and garlic and stir-fry for 3 minutes.

Add tomato paste and spices and cook for a further 3 minutes.

Add stock and water, coriander, parsley and tomatoes plus all hard vegetables.

Cover & cook for about 20 minutes, then turn down heat and simmer.

Add soft vegetables and cook until tender Serve on warm couscous sprinkled with sunflower seeds and pine nuts.

Serves 6-8

Fish Fillets with Couscous (Stage 3)

14oz (400g)	Fresh white fish fillets (ensure free of bones)
1 cup	Couscous
1 cup	Boiling vegetable stock
12	Green beans
1	Red capsicum (bell pepper), sliced
¼ cup	Pine nuts, toasted
2 tbsp	Parsley, chopped
6	Black olives halved

Preparation

Warm olive oil in pan and add fish and cook.

Place couscous into a bowl and pour over boiling stock.

Cover and leave for 5 minutes.

Cook beans and bell pepper until just tender.

Fluff up couscous with a fork Add pine nuts, parsley, olives and vegetables.

Serve fish on top of couscous.

Serves 2

Tempeh with Chinese Greens & Noodles (Stage 3)

5 tbsp	Cold pressed olive oil
2 medium	Onions, cut into 8 pieces
3	Garlic cloves (optional)

17-18oz (500ml)	Vegetable Stock
1 tbsp	Freshly grated ginger
1	Birdseye chili, finely chopped (optional)
2 tbsp	Salted black beans, soaked in boiling water for ½ hour (optional)
6	Shiitake mushrooms, soaked in boiling water for 10 mins or until soft, keep mushroom liquid, and finely slice mushrooms
3 tbsp	Mirin (is a golden liquid made from brown rice) -optional
6 tbsp	Soy sauce or tamari
1 bunch	Bok choy
1 bunch	Choy sum (can be replaced with other green vegetables)
1 bunch	Gaii choy (Chinese mustard greens)
1 bunch	Chinese broccoli
1 head	Broccoli, wash, cut into small florets, including stalk
17-18oz (500g)	Fresh rice noodles, thick or thin
13-14oz (375g)	Tempeh, cut in half, then into thin slices
3 tbsp	Sunflower seeds, dry roasted
3 tbsp	Pine nuts or peanuts, toasted

If more convenient all the Asian greens in this recipe could be replaced with other green vegetables – green beans, broccoli, snow peas, spinach etc.

Preparation

Heat saucepan and add 3 tbsp oil and warm.

Add tempeh, cook for 2 minutes.

Sauté onion until soft and lightly brown.

Add garlic, ginger and chili, cook for three minutes.

Add drained beans and sliced mushrooms and stir.

Stir in 16oz of stock, with mirin, mushroom water and half the soy sauce/tamari.

Simmer for 10 minutes. Remove from heat and set aside.

Prepare the noodles.

Trim greens and wash very well.

Heat large fry pan, add 1 tbsp oil.

Toss in broccoli, till bright green.

Add greens, stems first, till wilted.

Toss in leaf ends, cook another 3 minutes.

Place on serving plate.

Reheat pan and add remaining oil and then rice noodles.

Cook on high heat until they soften and begin to brown and crisp on the bottom.

Add remaining soy, stock and cook for a further 3 minutes Remove from the heat, place on plate.

Pour hot black bean sauce over the greens and noodles.

Sprinkle seeds and nuts over the top.

Serves 6

Grilled Swordfish, Olive Tapenade & Garlic Mash (Stage 3)

6 fillets	Swordfish (can substitute flathead, blue eye cod, snapper or Atlantic salmon)
4.5oz (120g)	Black or green olive tapenade
8 large	Potatoes, peeled
2	Garlic cloves, peeled and finely chopped
1-2tbsp	Cold pressed olive oil
1 splash	milk

Freshly ground pepper and sea salt

Preparation

Chop potatoes into small chunks and place into saucepan of water, with chopped garlic and cook potatoes until soft.

Heat a large fry pan and add some oil and the fish.

Cook fish until golden brown.

Drain water from the potatoes and garlic.

Mash potatoes and garlic and remaining oil.

Whip potatoes and garlic with a fork to fluff up.

Place potato mash on serving plate in the center.

Add fish to the top of the potato.

Scrape a thin layer of tapenade onto the fish.

Serve with a green salad and freshly steamed asparagus.

Serves 6

Miso with Silken Tofu   *(Stage 3)*

Note: silken tofu is very delicate, handle with care

¼ cup	Dried Arame
5 cups	Vegetable stock
½ packet	Buckwheat noodles (cooked as per instructions on the packet)
½	Leek, washed and cut into julienne strips
3 tsp	Miso
1 tsp	Ginger, finely grated
14oz (400g)	Silken tofu
1 cup	Fresh green beans, washed and thinly sliced
Gomasio to serve, sprinkle on to taste	

Preparation

Add the arame to cook with the noodles, then drain and set aside.

Bring stock to boil and add leek and beans and simmer 1 minute.

Remove from heat, add drained arame, noodles, miso and ginger.

Stir broth constantly to dissolve miso (do not boil miso).

Cut tofu into slices and lightly brown in ghee or butter, then divide between four warmed bowls.

Pour noodles and vegetables with the broth over the tofu Sprinkle with Gomasio or sesame seeds and finely chopped spring onions

Serve with a fresh salad of choice

Serves 4

Lentil Fritters *(Stage 3)*

2 tbsp	Cold pressed sesame oil
1	Onion, finely chopped
1 tsp	Ground coriander
1 tsp	Sea salt
1 cup	Red lentils washed and soaked in cold water for 15 mins
5oz (140ml)	Vegetable stock
4 tbsp	Spring onions, chopped roughly
1	Egg, beaten
1 pinch	Ground black pepper/white pepper

Hemp seeds for coating the fritters

Ghee or cold pressed olive oil for stir frying

Preparation

Heat sesame oil in a wok/frying pan.

Stir-fry onions for 2 mins, add coriander, salt and lentils, and cook for another 2 mins.

Add stock, simmer, stirring often for approx 5 minutes until the water is absorbed.

Leave to cool.

Add rest of the ingredients to cooled lentils, mix well.

Heat oil for stir-frying in either a wok or small saucepan.

Coat the fritters in hemp seeds.

Drop heaped tablespoons of lentil mix into oil – approx 1 minute each side.

Repeat until all mixture is gone.

Remove from oil with a slotted spoon, drain on absorbent paper.

Serve hot or cold with a big green salad and Gomasio, or steamed vegetable salad with tahini dressing.

These fritters are great in lunch boxes. *Makes approx 20 fritters.*

Calamari and Rice   (Stage 3)

20oz (550g) Squid cleaned and sliced into rings

1 ½ cups	*Long grain rice (basmati, jasmine)*
2 tbsp	*Cold pressed olive oil*
2	*Shallots, finely chopped*
2	*Garlic cloves, crushed*
1	*Cinnamon stick*
3	*Cardamom pods, preferably green*
5 tsp	*Sea salt*
2 ¼ cups	*Fish or vegetable stock*

Marinade

2 tbsp	Fresh lime juice
1 tsp	Lemongrass, finely chopped
1 tsp	Chiliies, (red or green) finely chopped (optional)
1 tsp	Parsley, finely chopped
2 cloves	Garlic, crushed
2 tbsp	Tamari or fish sauce
1 tbsp	Toasted sesame oil
1 bunch	Coriander, washed and finely chopped

Preparation

Mix all marinade ingredients in a bowl.

Place squid in marinade and leave for 15 minutes.

Heat olive oil in a saucepan and stir-fry all the rice ingredients (except the rice).

Cook for a further 3 minutes.

Add stock, bring to the boil.

Stir in the rice when the stock is boiling.

Turn down the heat, stir and bring to a simmer.

Simmer rice for 15 minutes, or until liquid has disappeared.

Cover saucepan with lid, leave on lowest heat for 10 minutes.

Drain squid and place on top of rice and cover.

Increase the heat a little and leave to cook for 1 to 2 minutes.

Remove pan from heat, leave covered, place on a wet folded tea towel and leave for 2 minutes.

Take off lid, stir the squid through, pick out cinnamon stick and cardamom pods.

Add coriander and stir through. Serve hot with wilted greens (see below) or a fresh garden salad. *Serves 4-6*

Hot Fish Curry   (Stage 3)

20oz (550g)	Cod steaks or monk fish fillets (or ask the fish man what fish is good for curry) cut into chunks
3oz (80ml)	Cold pressed olive oil or coconut oil
3 cups	Coconut milk, canned
2 cups	Fish stock
16oz (450g)	Small new potatoes, scrubbed and washed
Enough cooked rice for each bowl	

Curry paste

1	Onion, chopped
3	Garlic cloves, chopped (optional)
2" (5cm)	Lemongrass, chopped, outer leaves discarded
1" (2.5cm)	Galingale, peeled and chopped
2	Kaffir lime leaves, shredded
1 tsp	Ground black pepper
4-5	Red chiliies, de-seeded and chopped (optional)
1 tbsp	Coriander seeds, roasted
1 tbsp	Cumin seeds, roasted
½ tsp	Ground nutmeg
½ tsp	Ground turmeric
1 tbsp	Fish sauce
2 tbsp	Lemon juice
1 tsp	Sea salt

Preparation

Heat oil in a large saucepan.

Brown fish slightly in oil and set aside.

Place all ingredients for the curry paste with 4 tbsp of coconut milk into a blender, blend until smooth.

Pour the paste into the saucepan and bring to the boil, then simmer for 5 minutes.

Add rest of coconut milk and stock, bring almost to the boil.

Add potatoes and simmer uncovered for 20 minutes.

Place fish on top of curry and continue to simmer for another 10 mins.

Serve curry on top of warm or hot rice.

Do not thicken the sauce as the consistency should be like a soup

Serves 4 - 6

Stir-Fry Tempeh with Vegetables   (Stage 3)

1 tbsp	Toasted sesame seed oil
1 tbsp	Sunflower seeds
1 tbsp	Sesame seeds
3 tbsp	Cold pressed olive oil or ghee
1" knob	Fresh ginger, grated
1 large	Onion, halved and roughly sliced
1	Red chili, de-seeded and thinly sliced (optional)
½ head	Broccoli, washed and cut into florets
1 cup	Fresh or frozen peas
6 pieces	Lotus root, halved
1 cup	Fresh corn cut from 1 corn cob
2 handfuls	Fresh green beans, washed, topped and tailed
4 tbsp	Tamari or light soy
2 cups	Vegetable or chicken stock
13oz (375g)	Tempeh, halved length ways then thinly sliced
1 bunch	Fresh coriander
1 cup	Pumpkin, thinly sliced
Rice for four people	

Preparation

Heat olive oil in a wok or large fry pan.

Toss in ginger, chili and onion, stir-fry for 3 minutes.

Add tempeh and cook until golden brown, stirring fairly constantly.

Add a splash of stock if you need to.

Toss in half of coriander and all the vegetables.

Pour in stock and tamari.

Continue to cook on a high heat until vegetables are cooked, with a little bit of crunch.

Pour toasted sesame seed oil over vegetables and stir through.

Turn off heat.

Serve in big deep bowls on top of rice – don't forget the delicious cooking juices for the rice.

Garnish with remaining coriander, sunflower and sesame seeds.

Serves 4

Vegetable Noodle Soup (Stage 3)

1 ½ bunches	English spinach, wash & remove large stalks, tear into pieces
½ bunch	Fresh coriander, wash & chop, including the roots
1 bunch	Fresh parsley, wash and chop, remove stems
½ bunch	Spring onions, washed and finely chopped
3.5oz (100g)	Fettuccine, broken into pieces
26oz (750g)	Red kidney beans or soybeans, (canned) drained

1 cup	Green lentils, cooked until tender (or you can use a can of lentils)
53oz (1½ ltr)	Vegetable or chicken stock
2	Brown onions, peeled and finely chopped
3 tbsp	Cold pressed olive oil
1 cup	Cooked rice
2 handfuls	Pine nuts, toasted

Preparation

Stir-fry brown onions until crisp in one tbsp cold pressed oil, set aside.

Mix spinach, coriander, parsley and spring onions together, set aside.

Heat 2 tbsp cold pressed oil in a large saucepan.

Place fettuccine, kidney beans, 1 cup of stock, cooked lentils and garlic into the large saucepan, cook for 5 minutes.

Pour in enough stock to cover the ingredients in the pan, cover and bring to the boil

Reduce heat and simmer for 15 minutes or until cooked.

Add greens and stir, allowing them to wilt, then add rice and cooked onions.

Simmer gently for 5 minutes.

Serve in large bowls, garnished with crisp onions and pine nuts.

Serves 6-8

Rice, Mung Dal, Cauliflower & Peas (Stage 3)

1 cup	Basmati rice
1 small	Cauliflower, washed, dried and cut into small florets
2 tbsp	Cold pressed olive oil or coconut oil

½ tbsp	Fresh grated ginger
½ tbsp	Hot green chili, de-seeded, finely chopped (optional)
1 tbsp	Cumin seeds
5oz (150g)	Moong dal, split, without skins (or red lentils, rinsed)
6oz (180g)	Fresh peas (or you can use frozen peas - defrosted)
7 cups	Vegetable stock
1 ½ tsp	Turmeric
2 handfuls	Almond flakes
1 pinch	Sea salt

Preparation

Wash rice until the water runs clear, generally about six rinses.

Heat oil in a large saucepan, add ginger, chili and cumin seeds, stir fry until the cumin seeds turn brown, stir constantly

Toss in the cauliflower, quickly, stir through and cook for a further 5 minutes.

Stir in the rice and dal (or lentils) and cook for another minute.

Pour in the fresh peas, stock and turmeric, bring to the boil.

Reduce heat to low, partially cover and cook slowly for 1 ½ hours, stir occasionally – cook until rice and dal are soft (cooking time will be less for lentils) – similar to porridge in consistency. If you are using frozen peas, add during the last 5 minutes of cooking time.

Stir frequently to stop sticking, before serving, add salt.

Serve in bowls garnished with flaked almond.

Serve with a large green salad drizzled with a tart dressing (such as oil and fresh lemon juice). *Serves 4 to 6*

Rice and Bean Hot Pot   (Stage 3)

17-18oz (500g)	Red or white kidney beans or soybeans, soaked over night
2	Celery stalks and leaves, washed and halved
3	Bay leaves, fresh if possible
4	Parsley sprigs
2 tbsp	Olive oil
17-18oz (500g)	Brown onions, chopped
5	Garlic cloves, crushed
2	Fresh chiliies, fresh (optional)
2	Tomatoes, chopped
2	Red capsicums (bell peppers), cored, de-seeded and very finely chopped
1 tbsp	Sweet paprika
1 bunch	Mint, parsley and coriander (altogether), chopped finely
1 handful	Fresh walnuts dry roasted, crushed
½ handful	Fresh pine nuts dry roasted
½ handful	Sesame seeds, toasted
Extra mint leaves for garnish	
Cooked rice for each plate	
Kitchen string	

Sauce

28oz (800g)	Tomatoes (may used canned), chopped
2 tsp	Cold pressed olive oil
½ bunch	Fresh parsley, finely chopped

Preparation - Beans

Boil the beans in water for 10 minutes, drain and discard the water.

Tie parsley, celery and bay leaves together.

Cover the beans with fresh cold water, add the herbs and simmer for 1 hour until the beans are just tender.

Drain beans and keep the cooking liquid and discard the herbs.

Preparation - Sauce

Empty tomatoes and their juice into a saucepan.

Add oil and parsley, simmer uncovered for 20 minutes, until thicker.

Heat oil in heavy casserole dish.

Add onions, garlic, chili, peppers, tomatoes and paprika, cook gently for approx 5 minutes.

Stir in the beans, the sauce and enough of the cooking liquid to cover the beans Season with salt and pepper, cover and cook in a pre-heated oven (150°C/300°F) for 30minutes, stir occasionally.

Add the mint, parsley and coriander, stir through.

Place warm rice in bottom of serving bowls.

Serve beans on top of the rice.

Garnish with dry roasted nuts and sesame seeds and a few mint leaves.

Serves 8

You may freeze remainder in individual containers for another day.

Sweets, Treats and Desserts

Coconut Custard   (Stage 2)

2 cups	Unsweetened coconut milk
1 tsp	Butter or ghee or coconut oil
2	Whole eggs
¼ tsp	Nature Sweet Natural Sugar Substitute (or to taste) or 1 tsp honey
1 tsp	Nutmeg, grated
½ tsp	Vanilla extract, or 1 vanilla bean

Preparation

Warm coconut milk and beat in the butter, ghee or oil.

In a separate bowl, beat eggs until frothy then add the Nature Sweet Natural Sugar Substitute or honey.

While still beating, add the warm milk in a thin stream.

Add vanilla.

Pour the mixture into a greased baking dish.

Place in shallow pan of water.

Bake at 300°F/160°C for 40 minutes until custard is set.

This custard is nice with baked or stewed fruits.

Serves 2 - 4

Apple and Pear Ice cream   (Stage 2)

1	Pear, stem removed, cored, skin off
1	Granny smith apple, cored, skin off
½ cup	Milk - Coconut, dairy or almond, sugar free
¼ tsp	Nature Sweet Natural Sugar Substitute or 1 tsp honey

2 tbsp	Plain full fat yoghurt
1 tbsp	Gelatine, or agar agar
15oz (425ml)	Coconut milk

Preparation

Mix all ingredients together in a food processor or blender, until smooth,

Pour into a container of your choice and freeze,

Serve in scoops with crushed almonds or with poached pears,

Serves 4

Banana Pops   (Stage 2)

Cool and delicious on a hot day. Large strawberries can be prepared the same way.

2	Passion fruit – scrape out the pulp
1 cup	Natural full fat sugar free yoghurt (soy, coconut or dairy)
4	Bananas, ripe but firm

Chopped nuts, hemp seeds or LSA to sprinkle

Preparation

Peel bananas, cut in half crossways.

Push a pop stick or bamboo skewer through center of banana.

Place in freezer until frozen hard.

Mix passion fruit pulp with yogurt and dip frozen bananas into mixture until covered, allow to drip drain.

Sprinkle with chopped nuts, seeds or LSA and return to freezer.

Makes 8 pops

Light and Lovely Bananas (Stage 2)

4 large	Bananas, peeled, sliced lengthways then crosswise
1 cup	Orange juice, freshly squeezed
½ cup	Lemon juice, freshly squeezed
1 tbsp	Orange rind or zest
1/8 tsp	Nature Sweet Natural Sugar Substitute or 1 tsp honey
1 tsp	Cinnamon
3	Passion fruit (pulp only)

Preparation

Place juices, sweetener and orange rind in a large flat pan and heat until it simmers.

Add cinnamon, then add sliced bananas and cook for 1 to 2 minutes

Remove immediately to serving comport Spoon over juices and top with passion fruit

Serves 4

Cantaloupe (Rock Melon) Pops (Stage 2)

½   Cantaloupe or Rock Melon

1 cup   Natural full fat plain yogurt

½ cup Pineapple in natural juice, drained or fresh, diced (juice not required)

1 tsp   Fresh mint, finely chopped

Chopped nuts or LSA for sprinkles

Preparation

Peel and de-seed half a cantaloupe or rock melon.

Cut cantaloupe or rock melon into wedges of similar size to half a banana.

Place a pop stick or bamboo skewer into wedges and freeze.

Mix all remaining ingredients together.

Dip frozen cantaloupe or rock melon into mixture until covered, allow to drip drain.

Sprinkle with chopped nuts or LSA.

Return to the freezer. *Serves 2*

Berry Surprise   (Stage 2)

1 cup	Fresh raspberries, blackberries and/or loganberries
¼ tsp	Nature Sweet Natural Sugar Substitute or 1 tsp honey
1	Orange – grate rind and then juice orange
2 tsp	Gelatine, dissolved in a little hot water (or agar agar)
1 cup	Natural full fat plain yogurt

Preparation

Warm berries, sweetener, rind and juice in a small saucepan over low heat.

Add gelatine mixture and stir. Allow to cool.

Gently fold yogurt through berry mixture.

Place in 4 individual serving dishes.

Chill in refrigerator.

Serve garnished with a few extra berries or sliced kiwi fruit.

Serves 3

Rhubarb   (Stage 2)

This is tasty served with fresh cream or natural yoghurt.

8-9 oz (250g)	Fresh rhubarb, washed trimmed and cut into pieces
1 cup	Water
½ tsp	Nature Sweet Natural Sugar Substitute or 1 tsp honey
1	Fresh banana

Preparation

Cover rhubarb with water, add sweetener and slowly bring to the boil.

Simmer for 2 to 3 minutes.

Remove from heat, cool, then add sliced banana.

Serve with muesli for breakfast, or with yogurt for dessert.

Serves 2

Dried Pear Delights   (Stage 2)

17-18oz (500g)	Dried pears, minced
2 tsp	Powdered ginger
2 tsp	Powdered cinnamon
½ cup	Fresh lemon juice or fresh orange juice
9oz (250g)	Smooth nut spread (such as ABC Melrose)
½ cup	Desiccated coconut
	Whole almonds or cashews

Preparation

Mix all ingredients together, except whole nuts, until well combined and firm.

Take a whole nut and cover with mixture, and roll into a ball.

Can use extra coconut, when rolling, if mixture is sticky.

Repeat until all mixture is used.

Store in airtight container in fridge. Will keep for months if frozen.

Note: Lovers of ginger may use minced preserved ginger for stronger flavor.

Option: Substitute dried pears with dried apricots for variety.

Stewed Fruits in Season *(Stage 2)*

Use whatever fruits are in season. Apples, pears, peaches or nectarines. In winter, I love the black plums.

8	*Black plums, cut in half and pitted*
1	*Cinnamon stick*
2	*Cloves*
1 tsp	*Vanilla*
½ - 1 tsp	*Nature Sweet Natural Sugar Substitute or 1 tsp honey*
¼ cup	*Water*

Freshly grated nutmeg

Preparation

Place all ingredients in a saucepan. Bring to the boil and then gently simmer for 15 – 20 mins with the lid on.

Serve with plain yoghurt or fresh cream.

Serves 4

Oatmeal Pie Crust *(Stage 3)*

2 cups	*Rolled oats*
1 cup	*Hot water*
½ cup	*Rice flour*
1 tbsp	*Cold pressed olive oil*
1 tbsp	*Lemon juice*

Preparation

Mix oats and water and bring to the boil in a saucepan, stirring constantly until mixture thickens.

Stand until cold. Fold in the other ingredients and press mixture into a pie dish or 2 small pie dishes. Fill with your favorite filling.

For sweet filling add 1 tbsp honey or ¼ to ½ tsp Nature Sweet Natural Sugar Substitute. For savory filling add salt or herbs to taste.

American Pumpkin Pie   (Stage 3)

2 cups	Pumpkin (butternut/blue) – cook, mash and drain
1 cup	Soft tofu
1 ½ tsp	Cinnamon
½ tsp	Ground ginger or freshly grated ginger
½ tsp	Ground nutmeg
¼ cup	Rice, oat or almond milk
½ tsp	Nature Sweet Natural Sugar Substitute or 1 tsp honey
1 tbsp	Orange rind grated
½ cup	Pecans or walnuts, chopped

Preparation

Blend all ingredients except nuts, in a food processor until smooth.

Pour mixture into 23cm (9-inch) pie dish, lined with uncooked pie crust.

Sprinkle top with nuts.

Bake at 160°C/320°F for 35 to 40 minutes until golden and set.

Garnish with any fresh fruit – kiwi fruit looks nice. Serve with next best cream if desired. Serves 4

Next Best Cream   (Stage 3)

A non-dairy, gluten free cream, great on fresh fruit or fruit cooked in natural juices only.

7oz (200g)	Silken tofu
1 cup	Unsweetened coconut milk (canned)
¼ tsp	Nature Sweet Natural Sugar Substitute or 1 tsp honey
½ tsp	Pure vanilla essence
3 tbsp	Arrowroot

Preparation

Blend arrowroot with a little coconut milk in a saucepan.

Add remaining milk.

Stir continually over a medium heat until the mixture thickens.

Allow to cool. Add all other ingredients to thickened mixture.

Beat with an electric mixer on low speed until mixture is thick and resembles whipped cream.

Serve with fresh fruit or anywhere that you would use cream.

Serves 4.

Carrot and Apple Cake   (Stage 3)

1 cup	Wholemeal SR flour or buckwheat or spelt flour
1 tsp	Nature Sweet Natural Sugar Substitute or 1 tsp honey
¾ cup	Pecans or walnuts, chopped
1 cup	Carrot, grated
1 cup	Granny smith apple grated, leave on skin
2 tbsp	Cocoa or Cacao powder
½ tsp	Bicarb soda
2	Eggs, whole

Preparation

Sift flour, cocoa and soda into large bowl.

Mix in beaten eggs and all other ingredients and combine well

Spoon mixture into a greased ring tin.

Bake in a moderate oven for 40 - 45 minutes or until cooked.

Test with a skewer, cool in tin Serve dusted with a little cinnamon.

Syndrome X Energy Slice   *(Stage 3)*

This slice is unbelievably tasty, nutritious and energy boosting.

1 cup	Natural sultanas
½ cup	Dates, chopped
½ cup	Dried nectarines, chopped
1 cup	Dried apricots, chopped
1 cup	Mixed nuts chopped – almond, cashews, Brazil or pecans
½ cup	Sunflower seeds
½ cup	Pepitas
3 cups	Freshly squeezed orange juice
1 tsp	Mixed spice

Put all ingredients in a saucepan and heat slowly until just simmering.

Remove from heat to cool.

When cool, put into a large bowl with –

¾ cup	LSA
1 ½ cups	coconut, buckwheat or hemp flour
2 large	Eggs, whole, beaten

Spread evenly into a baking pan lined with baking paper.

Sprinkle top with -

¼ Cup   Sesame seeds

Press seeds down firmly and bake in medium oven at 150°C/300°F for 45 minutes to one hour, or until cooked when tested with skewer

Cool in tin.

Using a sharp knife cut into fingers and store in airtight container.

Note: Brazil nuts are ideal for this recipe and provide extra selenium.

Tangy and Spicy Apple Bake   (Stage 3)

2 large	Green apples, peeled and cored
3 tbsp	Lemon or orange juice
1 tsp	Lemon or orange rind, grated
1 tsp	Nature Sweet Natural Sugar Substitute or 1 tsp honey
1 tbsp	Raisins or natural sultanas
8	Dried apricots
8	Prunes, pitted
½ tsp	Cinnamon, ground
½ tsp	Grated nutmeg

Preparation

Slice apples into thin wedges.

Toss in juice and arrange wedges around the edge of a casserole dish.

Combine the juices with the rind, Nature Sweet and dried fruits. Sprinkle through the cinnamon.

Place this mixture through the center of the casserole.

Cover with foil.

Bake at 320°F/160°C for 30 minutes or until apple is tender. Serve warm, topped with fresh cream or natural yoghurt.

This dish can be prepared a few hours ahead and warmed before serving.

Serves 4

Baked Winter Fruit Salad   *(Stage 3)*

2 large	Green apples, peeled and thinly sliced
2 large	Pears, peeled and thinly sliced
1 tsp	Cinnamon, ground
½ tsp	Grated nutmeg
¼ tsp	Nature Sweet Natural Sugar Substitute or 1 tsp honey
½ cup	Raisins, seeded
½ cup	Almonds, blanched and sliced
1 tbsp	Orange peel, shredded
1 small tin	Unsweetened crushed pineapple, drained, keep juice

Preparation

Mix together pineapple, sweetener, raisins, cinnamon and peel.

Place 1/3 of apples and pears overlapping, in a deep 23cm (9-inch) pie dish.

Top with ½ of the mixture.

Place another 1/3 layer of apple and pear slices.

Top with remaining half of mixture.

Finish with the apple and pear layer.

Pour remaining pineapple juice over the fruit.

Cover dish and bake in a moderate oven for 45 minutes

Remove cover, shake a little extra cinnamon and nutmeg over top and sprinkle the almond slices Serve warm with a dollop of next best cream.

Serves 6.

Pear Truffles   (Stage 3)

Serve these with coffee after a leisurely dinner

1 cup	Pears, dried
¾ cup	Raisins
1 tsp	Preserved ginger (more if desirable)
1 tsp	Nature Sweet Natural Sugar Substitute, 1 pinch stevia or 1 tsp honey
1 tbsp	Fruit juice (apple or orange)
1 tbsp	LSA
1 cup	Shredded coconut, toasted

Preparation

Mince dried fruit and ginger

Combine in a bowl with sweetener, fruit juice, LSA and ½ of the coconut.

Mix well Form mixture into small balls and roll in the remaining coconut.

Slightly flatten to form thick button shapes.

Refrigerate until firm then store in fridge in an airtight container.

Can be made several days ahead.

Fruity Petit Fours   (Stage 3)

1 cup	Dried pears, chopped
½ cup	Dried apricots, chopped
½ cup	Cashews, chopped

½ cup	Shredded coconut
1 tbsp	Lemon juice
1 pinch	Nature Sweet Natural Sugar Substitute or stevia
5oz (425ml)	Coconut cream, unsweetened

Preparation

Mix all ingredients together with enough coconut cream to bind the mixture.

Stand covered for 1 hour.

If mixture is too dry, add more coconut cream to hold it together and make it pliable.

Roll into small balls.

Press a cashew nut into top of each ball.

Place in small confectionery paper-patty cups.

Cover and store in fridge in an airtight container.

Peachy Treats   (Stage 3)

Made in a flash, this dessert is light and very tasty

Peach or pear halves can be used

30oz (825g)	Peach halves, drained or 6 - 8 fresh peaches
3½oz (100g)	Natural plain full fat yogurt or coconut yogurt
1 cup	Mixed dried fruit, chopped
1 tbsp	Apple or orange juice
1 pinch	Ground cinnamon
½ cup	Toasted coconut

Preparation

Arrange peach halves in individual serving dishes.

Mix fruit juice with dried fruit.

Stand for about ½ hour, then fold into yogurt.

Spoon mixture into hollows of peaches, sprinkle with cinnamon.

Top each serve with coconut.

Serves 6 to 8.

Banana Cake   (Stage 3)

9oz (250g)	Wholemeal SR flour or spelt flour or buckwheat flour
½ cup	Cold pressed oil
2 tsp	Nature Sweet Natural Sugar Substitute, 3 pinches stevia or 1 tsp honey
2 large	Ripe bananas, mashed
3 tbsp	Milk – A2 dairy, soy, oat or coconut
1 tsp	Bicarb soda
1 tsp	Vanilla extract, or 1 vanilla bean
2	Eggs

Preparation

Beat oil and sweetener until smooth, add eggs and beat well.

Add mashed bananas, mix in milk, bicarb soda and vanilla together.

Add alternately with sifted flour until all ingredients are folded smoothly together.

Place mixture in a lined cake tin.

Sprinkle with cinnamon or chopped walnuts.

Cook in a moderate oven for about 45 minutes, test with skewer.

Cool in tin for 10 minutes before removing to a cooling rack.

Poached Fruitee Pears   (Stage 3)

3 large	Pears, peeled and cored
½ cup	Dried apricots, chopped
½ cup	Shredded coconut
¼ cup	Almonds, chopped
½ tsp	Cinnamon
1 tsp	Nature Sweet Natural Sugar Substitute or 1 pinch stevia (if desired)
1 cup	Apple or apricot juice, unsweetened

Preparation

Cut pears in half and lay centre-up in a casserole dish.

In a bowl, mix together apricots, coconut, almonds and cinnamon.

Add enough Nature Sweet to taste.

Divide the mixture evenly over the six pear halves. Add one cup of juice to casserole, pour over the fruit.

Cover and bake in preheated oven at 350°F/180°C, approx 30 minutes.

Serve warm, with apple and pear ice cream, or fresh cream.

Serves 4 or more.

Apple Crumble   (Stage 3)

Pie Filling ingredients:

6 – 8	Apples
1½ tsp	Vanilla extract, or 1 vanilla bean
350ml (12oz)	Water
1 - 2 tsp	Cinnamon

Custard ingredients:

17oz (500ml)	Coconut Cream or Dairy milk
2½ tbsp	Xanthan gum or arrowroot
2½ tbsp	Coconut sugar or 1 teaspoon honey or ½ teaspoon of Nature Sweet Sugar Substitute
2 tsp	Vanilla extract

Crumble Ingredients:

¾ oz (20g)	LSA
1 cup	Macadamias, ground
5oz (140g)	Almond meal
1 tsp	Cinnamon
1 tsp	Nutmeg
2½oz (70g)	Coconut sugar or 2 tbsp honey
½ cup	Coconut oil
2 tbsp	Arrowroot - Xanthan gum is also an option to thicken
1 Cup	Fresh or frozen berries

Preparation

Preheat oven to 350 F/180 C.   Wash and remove the apple core and cut into wedges with the skin left on (optional). Place the apples into a large saucepan with water, vanilla and cinnamon and cook over medium to low heat for about 20 – 30 minutes, stirring occasionally until the apples have completely softened. Cover for half of the cooking time.

Crumble: Combine almond meal, LSA, ground macadamias, cinnamon, nutmeg, arrowroot and coconut sugar in a bowl. Stir to combine. Add coconut oil using your fingertips, rub into dry ingredients until mixture resembles coarse breadcrumbs.

Place apples into a heatproof pie dish or 6 – 8 individual ramekins and add berries.

Pour custard over the apples then sprinkle crumble over custard.

Bake for 40 minutes or until golden. Serve warm with plain full fat yoghurt or coconut ice cream.

Making the custard: Mix the arrowroot or custard powder, coconut sugar and 3 tablespoons of water in a saucepan until smooth on medium to high heat, then slowly add the almond milk while stirring until it boils. Then reduce the heat and let it simmer for 1 minute. Then remove from heat and let it stand, this will thicken the custard.

Alternatives

Apples – peaches, pears

Almond meal – cashew meal, macadamia meal

Healthy Chia Balls (Stage 2)

Chia Chews are full of wholefoods that will strengthen your energy systems- unlike highly processed sugary foods. The natural sugars of our Chia Chews will give you long lasting energy that won't leave you feeling drained like the slump that follows a refined sugar spike.

Cherries are known to alkalize the body- assisting with relief of painful gout caused by a build up of uric acid. Cherries are full of anti oxidants and even contain the sleep inducing hormone- Melatonin!

These balls are full of fibre to reduce constipation and are high in Omega 3 fats (from Chia and Flaxseeds) with a load of crunchy texture from macadamias nuts. These balls are full of nutrition that your body will love you for- and they taste great!

Amounts of ingredients do not have to be exact – vary according to your taste

4oz (120g)	Macadamia nuts
5oz (150g)	Tart dried cherries
4 tbsp	Chia seeds
6	Dried Figs
2 tbsp	Coconut oil
1 tbsp	Vanilla extract
1 tbsp	Ground ginger
1 tsp	Ground cinnamon
1 tsp	Sea salt

Directions

Place figs, nuts, chia seeds and cherries in a food processor, blend until well ground. You may need to scrape the sides. Slowly blend in vanilla, ginger, cinnamon, coconut oil and salt. Remove mixture from food processor. Roll into balls and wrap in small brown paper bags or other wrap.

Serving Size: 12 individual balls. As a snack do not eat more than 2 at a time, as figs are high in sugar

Low Carb (Paleo) Banana Bread   (Stage 2)

Sugar free, grain free.

If you want to put a name to it- Banana Bread Paleo style!

Thanks to it being cane sugar free, with its low carbohydrate and high fibre content- this is a recipe that even a diabetic can enjoy in moderation.

Coconut flour has the highest fibre content of any other flour- which assists not only weight management, but keeping blood sugar levels low. High in Protein- in fact 20% protein, coconut flour contains essential amino acids. This is a wholesome nutritious treat, it won't taste like your sugar laden banana bread from the local cafe - it will taste better! If you really need a bigger sugar hit - I have added some options at the bottom of this recipe.

Ingredients

4 medium Bananas - mashed

They can be yellow- but this is a great opportunity to use your older black speckled skinned bananas that even the possums turn their nose up at.

4	*Organic Eggs, whisked*
1 cup	*Coconut flour*
½ cup	*Macadamia Butter (Macadamia was my choice, however you can use almond butter, coconut butter- whatever nut or seed butter you prefer.)*
4 tbsp	*Dairy butter, softened*
1 ½ tbsp	*Cinnamon*
1 tsp	*Baking Soda*
1 tsp	*Baking Powder (Gluten free)*
1 ½ tsp	*Organic Vanilla Bean extract.*

Method:

Preheat your oven to 170°C (340°F).

Combine your bananas, eggs, nut butter and organic butter. Mix well using a food processor- even your regular electric hand beater will do the job.

Once all of your ingredients are blended, add in your coconut flour, cinnamon, baking soda, baking powder, vanilla and mix well.

Grease a regular sized loaf tin with the fat of your choice - I use butter. 10"x 4"x 2½" (25x10x7cm) is approx your average sized tin. It will bake in approx 35-40 mins- but ovens can vary, so keep an eye on it.

Stick a skewer into the center. If it comes out clean- it's ready.

Remove from oven and flip straight out onto a cooling tray.

Slice and serve hot with a little dairy butter or tahini.

Homemade banana bread goes well with any one of the following combos!

Dairy butter with crushed macadamias and honey

Coconut syrup and cinnamon

Coconut butter and cinnamon - options are endless!

Coconut Baked Apples   *(Stage 3)*

Ingredients

4	Large apples
¾ cup	Coconut syrup
½ cup	Walnuts
¼ Cup	Raisins
2 tbsp	Dairy butter, cut into pieces
Cinnamon	

Serve with full fat plain yogurt

Directions

Heat oven to 200 degrees Celsius (390 degrees Fahrenheit).

Remove the apple cores and trim about a ½ inch (1cm) slice from the bottom of each apple, so they sit flat. Place the apples in an ovenproof dish.

Drizzle the apples with the syrup. Divide the walnuts and raisins among the apples, filling the cavities, and place any extra in the dish. Dot the apples with the butter. Bake until tender, 40 to 50 minutes.

If using a baking dish, pour the liquid from the dish into a skillet. Bring to a boil over medium heat. Cook until it thickens slightly, 2 to 3 minutes. Spoon the sauce over the warm apples, sprinkle with cinnamon and serve with yogurt if you chose.

Coconut syrup has a glycemic index in the low 30s- which makes it low on the Glycemic Index in comparison to Maple

Syrup which has a Glycemic index in the 50's. Coconut sugar also retains quite of bit of the nutrients found in the coconut palm. It also contains inulin, a fibre which slows glucose absorption; this explains its lower glycemic index.

Brownies made with beans and cherries (Stage 3)

1¾	Cups cooked black beans OR 1 can black beans, well rinsed
1½ Cups	Toasted Brazil nuts - see method on how to toast
2oz (60g)	80 to 90% cocoa chocolate
2 tsp	Chia seeds
4	Dates pitted
¾ Cup	Fresh or frozen cherries
4 tbsp	Cacao powder
2 tsp	Baking soda
1 tsp	Baking powder
¼ tsp	Cayenne
1 tsp	Cinnamon
½ tsp	Salt
1 tsp	Almond extract
5 drops	Oil of orange (optional)

10 drops of liquid stevia or 2 tbsp honey or 1 dessertspoon Nature Sweet Sugar Substitute.

Line a pan with baking paper and brush with coconut oil.

Preheat oven to 165 degrees Celsius (330 degrees Fahrenheit).

Toast 1½ cups of Brazil nuts for 10-15 min at 165 degrees Celsius (330°F). Pulse the nuts in a food processor to grind very coarsely, and reserve ¾ cup of ground Brazil nuts. Grind the rest until they become nut butter, which takes a minute or two. Scoop out and reserve. Put chopped dark chocolate in the processor, and grind until you've got fine pieces.

Add the rinsed beans, Chia seeds, sweetener, dates and cherries and process for 3-4 minutes. Add back the nut butter and the rest of your ingredients, except the reserved Brazil nuts, and process until smooth.

Mix Brazil nut chunks into the batter. Put the batter evenly into prepared pan. Bake 30 minutes then cover loosely with foil and continue to bake until a toothpick comes out clean, about 45-50 minutes.

Berry Pancakes *(Stage 3)*

Ingredients:

1	Cup buckwheat flour
1	Egg
1 Cup	Milk (dairy, almond or coconut milk)
2 tbsp	Coconut oil plus extra for pan
¼ Cup	Goji berries. Soaked in water and drained
½ Cup	Berries of choice
2 tsp	Honey or 1 tsp of Nature Sweet Sugar Substitute (optional)

Butter or cream (optional)

Method:

Whisk together egg, oil, milk and buckwheat, then add Goji berries and other berries.

Add a teaspoon of coconut oil to a pan and heat to medium heat.

Add your pancake batter to pan. Allow the batter to spread and cook until you can view holes developing on the top side- this is an indication the underside of the pancake is cooked.

Set cooked pancakes aside whilst cooking the remaining- be sure to cover them to keep the heat in.

Serve with cream (dairy or coconut)

What causes us to store fat?

Incorrect diet

In this day and age the food keeps getting faster and faster, and we are getting slower and slower!

When it comes to the cause of insulin resistance, the statement that "it is not how much you eat, but what you eat" is very true. The consumption of refined carbohydrates containing sugar and flour has produced the epidemic of insulin resistance we have in the developed world today.

We have evolved for hundreds of thousands of years, subsisting on a cave man's diet of meat, fish and vegetables and fruits – in other words food that is unprocessed and devoid of refined carbohydrates. The cave man diet is known as the Palaeolithic diet.

Heart attacks were not common at the start of the twentieth century, and in 1930, heart attacks caused only 3000 deaths in the United States. (REF. 5)

When we take a look at the diets of people who lived in the early 1900s, we find that the amount of fat in the daily diet was generally higher than it is today. The main types of fats eaten by those who lived in the early 1900s were butter, lard and tallow. According to modern day medical opinion, the consumption of such fats should have produced an epidemic of heart attacks and obesity, but it did not. This is because during this era people did not eat the trans-fatty acids, gluten flour and sugar that bulk up the processed foods we eat today.

In the early 1900s, the types of carbohydrates consumed were not refined, and consisted of unprocessed grains and cereals, unrefined flour and unrefined molasses. They did eat sugar, but not in the refined packaged and fast foods that we now find lining the supermarket shelves.

Today it is not uncommon for people to eat half to one pound of sugar every day. We also eat large amounts of gluten and partially hydrogenated vegetable oils that contain trans-fatty acids. Trans-fatty acids are completely unnatural and are widely found in the modern diet, so that they have replaced the natural essential fatty acids. It is the consumption of trans-fatty acids, as well as excessive amounts of refined carbohydrates, that have caused us to become fatter.

Weight Excess

Syndrome X is more common in those whose excessive weight accumulates in the upper body. This means the excess fat is found in the abdominal cavity and abdominal wall and the trunk. The fat may form rolls or spare tires around the chest and abdomen.

The rest of the body may be quite muscular and relatively free of fat. Thus Syndrome X is more common in those with the Android Body Type, also known as the apple shaped body type – see www.liverdoctor.com. However any Body Type can develop Syndrome X if they become overweight.

If you are overweight and you lose weight you will become less insulin-resistant. The good news is that you do not need to lose massive amounts of weight to reduce Syndrome X, and the typical over-weight individual can significantly reduce insulin resistance by losing only 10 kilograms (around 20 pounds).

Polycystic Ovarian Syndrome (PCOS)

Polycystic Ovarian Syndrome (PCOS) is a common hormonal imbalance in women, affecting around 10% of pre-menopausal women. PCOS often leads to an excess production of male hormones and a deficiency of progesterone. The term Polycystic Ovarian Syndrome is derived from the presence of small fluid filled sacs or cysts which accumulate in the ovaries from trapped eggs, which were never released from the ovaries. This is because normal ovulation (or release of the eggs) at the middle of the menstrual cycle is inhibited. Because ovulation does not occur regularly, these women do not produce adequate amounts of the hormone progesterone, which results in reduced fertility and irregular or very infrequent menstrual bleeding. Women with PCOS usually have higher levels of male hormones (androgens), which are produced in their ovaries, adrenal glands and also in their body fat. Weight excess will aggravate the hormonal imbalances of PCOS and is often associated with Syndrome X. The excess of male hormones will increase insulin resistance so that blood glucose problems result, especially in overweight women.

Overweight women with PCOS have a much higher risk of Syndrome X and a sevenfold increased risk of becoming a type 2 diabetic. Thus it is vital that they learn to control their weight and get their insulin levels down.

Although insulin-sensitizing medications such as Metformin can help those with PCO Syndrome, dietary changes remain the best strategy for long term success. Some women with PCOS are treated with the oral contraceptive pill, to give them a regular menstrual bleed and to "balance their hormones". However, long term use of the contraceptive pill, especially high dose pills, may aggravate insulin resistance leading to weight gain. It also increases the risk of liver and breast cancer.

The hormonal imbalance of PCOS can often be controlled very well with the use of natural progesterone and nutritional supplements. Natural progesterone is given in the form of lozenges or creams, in a dose of 30 to 100mg daily for 2 weeks in every month. Natural progesterone does not aggravate insulin resistance or increase weight, and may help to relieve many symptoms of PCOS. Useful supplements for women with PCOS are magnesium, chromium and the herbs bitter melon and gymnema. These are found in Glicemic Balance capsules. A good liver formula containing St Mary's Thistle, Taurine, selenium and B vitamins, such as LivaTone Plus, will help the liver to metabolize excessive estrogens and male hormones that are often found in overweight women with PCOS.

Genetic factors

Genetic factors are important in assessing your risk of Syndrome X. If you have a family history of obesity, diabetes type 2, hypertension, polycystic ovaries or heart disease, your risk of Syndrome X will be higher.

Lack of fitness

Insulin resistance is far more common in those who have a sedentary lifestyle and do not exercise regularly. Lack of fitness may increase your risk of Syndrome X by up to 25%. Although exercise reduces insulin-resistance, this benefit is lost if you stop exercising.

Medications

The chemical imbalance of Syndrome X can be accelerated by some drugs such as thiazide diuretics, high dose oral contraceptive pills, steroids such as body building hormones, cortisone, or the adverse effect upon the liver of taking too many prescribed medications. I have seen quite a few patients who have put on weight after commencing to take multiple medications, such as anti-inflammatory drugs, blood pressure drugs, cholesterol lowering drugs, anti-depressants and diuretics etc. Some people take as many as 7 to 8 different prescribed medications and their liver becomes very overworked having to break down all these drugs. Thus there is less energy left in the liver cells for burning fat. Weight gain then occurs.

As you can see, there are several factors that can play a role in the genesis of Syndrome X, which gives a researcher a profound respect for the complexity of this disorder. Although Syndrome X is complex, we now know how to overcome it. We do this with new nutritional strategies that make some of the previously so-called "healthy conventional diets" somewhat obsolete and ineffective. You may not be surprised by this statement, as I am sure that many of you will have found that conventional low-fat, high-carbohydrate diets did not work for you.

Triple strategy to burn fat

1. Reduce high insulin levels

2. Help insulin to work better

3. Improve your liver function

1. Reduce Insulin Levels

To lower insulin levels, we need to lower blood glucose (sugar) levels and keep them stable. If the blood glucose is persistently high, even if only slightly high, the pancreas will pump out larger amounts of insulin thus elevating blood insulin levels. If the blood glucose becomes excessively low, this causes the release of other hormones such as adrenalin and cortisol from the adrenal glands. These hormones cause the blood glucose to rise again, which will then stimulate the pancreas to pump out more insulin so that the blood glucose levels fall again. Thus the blood glucose levels go up and down precipitously, causing extreme cravings for sugar and carbohydrates and sometimes for alcohol. These cravings are very powerful, so that the sufferer becomes addicted to sugary foods and is unable to stay away from these problem foods.

My eating plan will stabilize the blood glucose levels, thus reducing the blood glucose highs and lows. This prevents high levels of insulin and other hormones such as adrenalin and cortisol. High levels of adrenalin and cortisol can elevate the blood pressure, cause anxiety, headaches, tremors and sweating. High levels of the hormone insulin make you very hungry so that you need larger amounts of food to feel satisfied. Some people with Syndrome X feel so hungry they could eat the door off the refrigerator!

Eating plan summary

Reduce refined carbohydrates

The most important carbohydrates to reduce are those that are refined and made from white sugar and white flour. Refined carbohydrates are those with a high Glycemic Index (GI). The Glycemic Index (GI) is a standard scale used to measure the ability of specific carbohydrate foods to elevate blood glucose levels. Pure glucose is used as the standard measure of the GI and is given the number of 100 on the GI scale. Foods with a lower number on the scale have a lower GI. For example lentils and beans are much lower on the GI scale than bread and sweets, while meat, eggs, seafood and poultry are virtually zero. See page 317 for more information on the Glycemic Index.

Foods that have a high GI number are typically refined or simple carbohydrates, and will quickly cause elevation of blood glucose and insulin levels, especially if they are eaten alone without protein or fat.

Refined carbohydrates are found in many highly processed breads and packaged cereals, cakes, biscuits and cookies, crackers, chips, pastry, some types of pasta, candies, milk chocolate, ice-cream, and packaged snack foods.

Your body has a limited ability to metabolize carbohydrates, and it will convert excess carbohydrates into body fat.

There are many versions of the popular high protein/low carbohydrate diet, and their carbohydrate content varies considerably. I recommend around 40% of your daily calories, come from complex carbohydrates, although in some people with very severe insulin resistance, carbohydrate intake will need to be reduced to 25% of total daily calories.

Tolerance to carbohydrates varies greatly between individuals, from 60 grams daily to 300 grams daily. This depends upon body weight, amount of exercise, and insulin metabolism, and some experimentation may be needed to determine what is best for you.

Refined carbohydrates should be eliminated. Refined carbohydrates stimulate the production of insulin much more than complex carbohydrates do. If the carbohydrates are complex they contain fiber and nutrients, which will slow down the rapid rise in blood glucose and insulin levels.

By limiting carbohydrate intake, we can increase fat burning to provide an efficient source of energy.

Eat first class protein with every meal

First class protein is found in the following food groups:

- All seafood: such as fish, shellfish, squid and octopus
- Poultry
- Meats: red and white
- Eggs (boiled, poached, scrambled, or omelette)
- Protein powder (whey protein has the highest protein content)
- Dairy products the best ones being cheese and plain yoghurt
- Combination of any 3, from the following 4 groups - legumes (beans, lentils, peas) with grains with nuts with seeds. If you do not eat 3 of these 4 groups at the SAME TIME, you will not be getting all of the essential amino acids at one meal.

By eating carbohydrates with some fat and protein at the same meal, we are able to reduce the rapid insulin-stimulating rise in blood glucose.

Refined carbohydrate foods stimulate the secretion of the fat producing hormone insulin, whereas non-carbohydrate foods, namely fats and proteins do not stimulate the production of insulin.

Eat some raw plant food with every meal

This includes all raw fruits and vegetables. A maximum of 2 pieces of fruit daily is allowed if you are overweight. An unlimited amount of green vegetables is allowed. Raw food increases fiber and improves digestion and provides the best source of antioxidants. The consumption of raw food with every meal is a good idea in those with Syndrome X, as raw foods contain natural vitamins and active enzymes to revitalize the sluggish metabolism. By eating more vegetables you will reduce your total consumption of calories and lower blood glucose and insulin levels.

2. Help insulin to work better

It is possible to help the body cells to respond better to insulin. We can achieve this by improving the sensitivity of the body cells to insulin. By doing this we will reduce the need for the pancreas to produce excess amounts of insulin, which will assist weight loss.

There are specific herbs and nutrients that have been proven to improve glucose and insulin metabolism. They may be taken individually or combined together in Glicemic Balance for a synergistic effect.

The most effective are a combination of the following-

Gymnema Sylvestre (GS)

According to several human clinical trials the action of the herb Gymnema Sylvestre can be beneficial in those with elevated blood glucose levels. High blood levels of glucose and excessive glycosylation of proteins (sugar damaging the proteins) appear to be corrected by Gymnema Sylvestre. It is postulated that the beneficial action of GS works by regenerating damaged beta cells in the pancreas. The beta cells produce insulin and are often damaged in diabetics. Gymnema also reduces cravings for sugar and refined carbohydrates.

Clinical trials of Gymnema Sylvestre used an equivalent of 400mg daily of the whole herb from a 5:1 extract of Gymnema Sylvestre. *(REF. 7)*

Bitter Melon

The herb Bitter Melon is also known as Momordica Charantia, or bitter gourd.

The fruit of this plant, which is a member of the Cucurbitaceae family, is a popular food in many Asian cultures. Clinical trials and laboratory experiments using an extract of the dried fruit or ground seeds of Bitter Melon, revealed its ability to lower blood glucose levels. These studies found that Bitter Melon reduces excessive blood glucose levels and improves glucose tolerance in type 2 diabetics.

The recommended daily dosage of Bitter Melon is an equivalent of 5 grams of the fruit powder using an 8:1 standardized extract. (REF. 8)

Chromium picolinate

Chromium is required for the healthy function of the insulin receptors, which are situated on the surface of the cells. This is very important for those with insulin resistance where the receptors malfunction, and become resistant to the action of insulin. In other words chromium helps the cells to communicate better with insulin, thereby facilitating the transfer of glucose from the blood stream into the cell to be used as cellular energy. Deficiency of chromium is common in those who have consumed a diet high in refined carbohydrates. In those with Syndrome X, I highly recommend a supplement, which contains chromium picolinate, to make insulin more efficient. It is difficult to get all the chromium you need from your diet, as the richest sources are Brewer's yeast and liver.

Chromium is a vital component of Glucose Tolerance Factor (GTF) which improves insulin function. Those who are deficient in chromium have difficulty in regulating blood glucose levels. Chromium deficiency may be associated with anxiety, fatigue, sugar cravings, excess hunger and glucose intolerance. Many people who supplement with chromium picolinate find that their craving for carbohydrates and sweets diminishes greatly. There have also been reports that chromium supplements can help the conversion of excess fat into lean muscle tissue.

Chromium picolinate has been shown to reduce insulin resistance, lower blood glucose levels by 18%, and glycosylated hemoglobin (abbreviated to HgbA1c or HB1Ac) by 10%. *(REF. 9 & 10)*

Chromium picolinate is a bioactive source of this essential mineral. The efficiency of chromium absorption is very low, but the picolinic acid in the Chromium Picolinate form, is a mineral transporter, which gets chromium into the muscle cells.

Results from a study in Beijing indicate that chromium may be efficacious in treating type 2 diabetes. The metabolic effects of chromium picolinate in this large study of type 2 diabetics were comparable to oral hypoglycemic (diabetic) drugs.

A randomized study in 1996 of 180 patients with type 2 diabetes, showed that chromium picolinate improved blood glucose and insulin levels and reduced glycosylated hemoglobin.

Lipoic Acid

Lipoic acid is a natural substance, which has been demonstrated to be effective in improving glucose utilization and reducing the glycosylation of proteins. When blood sugar sticks to proteins in cells this is called the glycosylation of proteins and this causes serious damage to the proteins. This damage causes many of the complications of diabetes such as neuropathy and kidney damage. It can also lead to dementia. We must prevent this destructive damage by lowering blood sugar levels.

Lipoic acid participates in the oxidative decarboxylation of pyruvate, which places it at the crux of the conversion of glucose into energy. Lipoic acid has repeatedly been shown to counteract insulin resistance in muscle tissue, and this is the major mechanism whereby it effectively lowers blood glucose levels. The potent antioxidant action of lipoic acid may be very useful in slowing the development of diabetic cataracts and neuropathy. Supplementation with lipoic acid provides substantial health benefits to those with Syndrome X, and also to both type 1 and 2 diabetics. Doses of lipoic acid range from 100 to 600mg daily. *(REF. 11)*

Carnitine fumarate

Carnitine is involved in fat mobilization, and when it is deficient, overweight persons often find it very difficult to get into the fat burning area of metabolism. In other words, they have difficulty beginning the breakdown of body fat, which is called the stage of lipolysis and ketosis. Carnitine can be described as the "shovel" that puts the fuel into the energy factories (mitochondria) inside the cells. Carnitine transfers fatty acids across the mitochondrial membrane to be used as fuel. Carnitine helps the utilization of ketone bodies for energy; ketones are often elevated in those on extremely low carbohydrate diets (ketogenic diets) or in poorly controlled diabetics.

It has been reported that supplemental carnitine can reduce total blood fats, especially triglycerides. Carnitine deficiencies may contribute to potentially dangerous elevations in triglycerides and cholesterol. *(REF. 12)*

Supplemental carnitine may increase the burn rate of calories from stored fat by enhancing the efficiency of fatty acid oxidation. The richest dietary sources of carnitine are red meats (lamb and beef). Vegetables, fruits and many cereals contain little or no carnitine.

Selenium

Selenium should be supplemented in those with Syndrome X, and in diabetics, because of its proven protective effects on cell membranes and genetic material. Selenium is the vital partner for glutathione to exert its antioxidant effects in the body and especially the liver. *(REF. 13)*

Minerals to improve blood sugar control

Magnesium, manganese and zinc are involved in multiple enzyme systems within the energy producing mitochondria. A diet high in carbohydrates, especially of the refined types, may cause depletion of minerals such as magnesium, manganese, selenium and zinc, which will slow down metabolism. Magnesium has been shown to reduce insulin resistance and I highly recommend that you take supplemental magnesium. Trace mineral deficiencies are not uncommon in those with Syndrome X, and will worsen glucose intolerance. *(REF. 14)*

Nutrients beneficial for blood glucose control include the following -

- Gymnema Sylvestre (5:1 standardized extract) 27.0mg equiv. to 133.3mg
- Bitter melon (8:1 standardized extract) 208.3mg equiv. to 1666.7mg
- Chromium picolinate 134mcg
- Lipoic acid 70mg
- Carnitine fumarate 150mg
- Selenomethionine 8.6mcg
- Magnesium aspartate 16.7mg
- Manganese chelate 3.3mg
- Zinc chelate 1.33mg

There are several types of supplements available which contain the above nutrients. They are also available combined together in the correct amounts, in the supplement called Glicemic Balance. Take one to two capsules of Glicemic Balance with every meal. If you need more information on blood sugar control, phone the Health Advisory Service in Phoenix on 623 334 3232 and in Australia on 02 4655 8855.

These nutrients are helpful for -

- Insulin resistance and diabetes type 2
- Unstable blood glucose levels, including high blood glucose levels (hyperglycemia) and low blood glucose levels (hypoglycemia)
- Difficult to control cravings for sugar and carbohydrates
- Weight excess in those with impaired glucose tolerance
- Fatty Liver

These nutrients will not interact adversely with insulin or oral hypoglycemic drugs, however the patient must be guided by his/her own health practitioner.

Insulin dependent diabetics must not stop their insulin medication. Diabetics on oral hypoglycemic drugs can only stop their medication with their own doctor's approval. Those taking the above supplements for the first time may notice that their blood glucose levels drop, which is desirable of course. If the drop causes any unpleasant symptoms eat some protein food – generally only a small snack is required.

Other nutrients to reduce Insulin Resistance

To increase the sensitivity of your cells to insulin you need to:

Improve the quality of the receptors on the cell membranes, which attach to the insulin molecule. Chromium picolinate can improve the communication of insulin with the cell receptor to lower blood sugar levels.

Magnesium can have a beneficial effect upon the sensitivity of the cell membranes to insulin, which means that magnesium supplements may reduce insulin resistance. Low magnesium levels have been associated with insulin resistance, high levels of insulin and blood glucose abnormalities.

Berberine is a natural extract that can be remarkably effective for people with insulin resistance and/or diabetes type 2. It can also help with weight loss. The dose of berberine is one to two 500mg capsules, twice daily.

Another way to increase the sensitivity of your cell membrane receptors to insulin is to ensure that your diet contains abundant amounts of healthy fats.

The following foods provide the beneficial fats you need for healthy cell membranes –

- Oily fish such as salmon, trout, herrings, mackerel, sardines and tuna, which also provide first class protein, as well as omega 3 fatty acids
- Raw nuts and seeds - hemp seeds, chia seeds, pumpkin seeds, sesame seeds. Whole flaxseeds (grind in a grinder or blender) to make a fine powder. You can add one tablespoon of this powder to your cereal, smoothies or desserts, to provide extra omega 3 essential fatty acids
- Coconut flesh, milk and oil
- Avocado flesh and oil

3. Improve your liver function

Surprisingly, most people with weight excess do not think it has much to do with their liver. Indeed we mostly think about the liver as an organ to filter the toxins out of the blood stream and make vital proteins for our body. Doctors are not taught at medical school that liver function has anything to do with weight control, and they generally only focus on the liver if it becomes diseased. However we need to think about the liver as a very strategic organ in our plan for weight control. The healthy liver regulates fat metabolism, and is the major fat burning organ in the body. The liver is also able to pump excess fat out of the body via the bile, so it is carried out of the body in the bowel actions.

Fatty liver

Many overweight people have a fatty liver, which is not burning fat efficiently. A fatty liver does the opposite of what it is programmed to do, and stores fat, becoming a warehouse for fat. Obviously a fatty liver is not able to burn fat efficiently, which makes it very difficult for you to lose weight.

A healthy liver is really just a big filter with many spaces containing blood. The spaces are separated by rows of liver cells called hepatocytes. These specialized liver cells remove the excess fat from the blood in the spaces and process it. However, if your liver is fatty, the liver cells are full of fat, and cannot remove enough fat from the blood in the spaces. Thus the blood remains full of fatty particles, which circulate around the body and deposit in your fatty areas. Thus a fatty liver makes it very hard for you to lose weight.

Because fatty liver is so common, it used not to be considered as a liver disease. However this attitude is changing, as we now know that fatty infiltration of the liver can impair liver function, cause liver inflammation, and may lead to cirrhosis or cancer of the liver. In severe cases of fatty liver a liver transplant may be required. Syndrome X is the most common cause of fatty liver. The condition of fatty liver is also known in medical terms as Non-Alcoholic Steatorrheic Hepatosis (NASH) or steato-hepatitis.

How to tell if you have a fatty liver

You may have some or all of the following problems:

- Accumulation of fat in the abdominal area
- A roll of fat around the upper abdomen; I call this the liver roll
- Inability to lose weight
- Abnormal blood fats: high LDL cholesterol and triglycerides, and low HDL cholesterol
- High blood pressure

Tests for Fatty Liver

An ultrasound scan of the liver will show that the liver has an abnormal texture with fatty infiltrations and streaks of fat.

Your liver enzymes may be elevated if the fat is causing liver inflammation. In the early stages your liver enzymes may not be elevated. This can be tested for with a simple blood test.

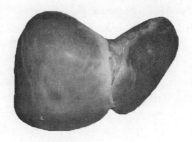

Healthy Liver

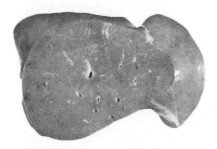

Fatty Liver

A fatty liver can be a toxic liver

Many environmental toxins and hormones are fat-soluble, and do not dissolve in watery fluids such as blood, bile and urine. These fat-soluble toxins can only be broken down by the liver cells, which contain enzymes to convert the fatty toxins into water-soluble forms. The liver cells perform this detoxification of fatty toxins via the step one and two detoxification biochemical pathways - see diagram. It is only possible for these fatty toxins to be eliminated from the body if they are converted to water-soluble waste products. Once they are water-soluble, these toxins can be eliminated from the body in watery fluids such as the bile, sweat, saliva and urine. If the liver is not able to perform its detoxification of these fatty toxins efficiently, these toxins will be deposited into the fatty areas of the body.

If you have a fatty liver, large amounts of these toxins can be deposited inside the fatty liver cells where they stagnate, and further compromise the metabolic processes of the liver cells. The fatty toxins will also be stored in other fatty areas of your body such as the brain, the hormonal glands, and fat deposits in the buttocks, abdomen, thighs, and indeed wherever you store fat.

These toxins can impair the inner metabolic processes of the fat cells so that your fat cells become sluggish and inactive. It is much harder to break down these toxic fat cells and indeed they often become cellulite.

This is why detoxification of the body can help with weight loss, as it helps to remove the toxins from the fat cells and liver cells. Once the toxins are removed the metabolic processes of the liver cells and fat cells are able to work much more efficiently, and normal fat metabolism is able to resume.

A fatty liver will cause problems with blood glucose control as it does not store glycogen as well as it should. Thus when your liver is called upon to release glucose into the blood stream from its glycogen stores, there is not enough to be released. Blood glucose levels then plummet and you start craving sugar again.

Symptoms that may be associated with Liver Dysfunction

- Blood glucose problems and insulin resistance
- Abnormalities in the level of fats in the blood stream, for example, elevated LDL cholesterol and reduced HDL cholesterol, and elevated triglycerides
- Arteries blocked with fat (atherosclerosis)
- Build up of fat in other body organs (fatty degeneration of organs)
- Lumps of fat in the skin (eg. lipoma and xanthelasma)
- Excessive weight gain and inability to lose weight
- Protuberant abdomen (pot belly) and/or a roll of fat

around the upper abdomen (Liver Roll)
- Cellulite
- Coated tongue and/or bad breath
- Skin rashes and/or itchy skin (pruritus)
- Excessive sweating and/or offensive body odor or overheating of the body
- Dark circles under the eyes, yellow discoloration of the eyes, and/or red swollen itchy eyes (allergic eyes)
- Acne rosacea - (red pimples around the nose, cheeks and chin) and a flushed facial appearance with excessive facial blood vessels
- Brownish spots and blemishes on the skin (liver spots)
- Red palms and soles, which may also be itchy and inflamed

NOTE: All of the above symptoms are common manifestations of a dysfunctional liver. However, they can also be due to other causes, of a more sinister nature, so, in all cases of persistent symptoms, it is vital to see your doctor.

How to improve your liver function

Think of yourself as a rabbit! This means that you need to start eating raw plant foods more regularly, especially salad vegetables. All varieties of vegetables may be used in salads and avocado is a great way to give a salad more body. Leafy greens, green herbs (such as parsley, basil, chives, coriander and mint etc), grated carrots and beetroot, cucumber, sprouts, shallots, onion, capsicums (bell peppers), and indeed any vegetable may be used: see our delicious salad recipes.

You should ideally eat some raw food with EVERY MEAL. It is quite OK to combine raw foods with cooked foods, as they improve digestion. It is generally beneficial to eat up to 3 to 4 pieces of raw fruit daily, unless you are overweight, when you will need to eat less. If you are trying to lose weight you may want to limit your pieces of fruit to no more than 2 daily until you have reached your desired weight. Many of my patients have told me that they only began to lose weight after they started to eat raw foods. They did not change their diet in any other way and were surprised to find that raw foods made all the difference. Raw foods stimulate the fat burning process, especially in the liver, because of their cleansing and anti-inflammatory effect upon the liver and lymphatic system.

Eat foods high in the mineral sulphur such as eggs, cruciferous vegetables (cabbage, Brussels sprouts, cauliflower, broccoli), and vegetables from the onion family, such as onions, leeks, shallots and garlic. Broccoli sprouts powder is very high in sulphur and can be purchased in most countries; try to get organic.

Sulphur helps the step two detoxification pathways of the liver to work more efficiently, and will promote weight loss and energy levels. An excellent supplemental source of organic sulphur to help the liver can be obtained by taking MSM, which stands for Methyl Sulphonyl Methane. MSM works better when combined with vitamin C. I recommend that you take half a teaspoon twice daily mixed in raw juices.

Start to juice regularly

Juices made freshly from raw vegetables have unique healing and rejuvenating properties on your liver and metabolism.

If you find the juices too strong, simply dilute them with water according to your taste. People with a weight problem should avoid juicing fruits, except for green apples, lemons, limes and grapefruits. Small amounts of orange juice or green apples may be added to moderate bitter or sour tastes. Generally speaking you should use 20% fruit and 80% vegetables in your juices.

Pure fruit juices (especially processed varieties) are high in fructose and sucrose, which will raise the blood glucose levels. If you are diabetic then it is better to avoid fruit juices and use only vegetable juices.

Juice for Syndrome X

This juice lowers insulin and blood sugar levels

> *½ cup green string beans, washed and ends cut off*
>
> *2 broccoli florets washed and sliced in half*
>
> *3 Brussels sprouts: washed and base cut off*
>
> *1 carrot*

Wash well and then pass all through the juicer; dilute 50% with water if desired and drink.

This combination can be effective in lowering blood glucose levels and improving liver function. This juice recipe will be helpful for weight loss if you have Syndrome X. If you cannot cope with the somewhat bitter taste, add a red apple to the juicer.

Liver Cleansing Juice

> *One carrot*
>
> *One cup cut cabbage*
>
> *One clove garlic (may reduce amount if it is too strong)*
>
> *One red radish*
>
> *1 lime or lemon*
>
> *¼ inch (½ cm) fresh ginger root*
>
> *1 green apple*

Pass all the above through the juicer. Take with 1tsp Livatone Plus powder

For more information and recipes on juicing, see my book titled *"Raw Juices Can Save Your Life"*

The liver plays a vitally important role in the regulation of carbohydrate metabolism and blood glucose control.

The liver manufactures a substance called glucose tolerance factor (GTF), which helps insulin to work more efficiently.

The liver stores glycogen and contains approximately 80 grams of glycogen. When blood glucose levels drop, such as in between meals, the liver breaks down the glycogen into glucose and releases the glucose into the blood stream. This prevents the blood glucose level from dropping too low and maintains a stable level of blood glucose.

It manufactures glucose by a process called gluconeogenesis. The raw materials that the liver uses to synthesize glucose are lactate, pyruvate, amino acids (mainly alanine and glutamine), and glycerol from the breakdown of fat stores.

The liver plays a vitally important role in fat metabolism, which is important in the development of Syndrome X and obesity.

To put it simply one could say that the liver is the major fat burning organ in the body. It manufactures fats, recycles fats, and pumps excessive fats out of the body through the bile into the intestines.

The fats called cholesterol and triglyceride are manufactured in the liver. Cholesterol is the raw material for the body's production of natural steroid hormones, sex hormones and vitamin D and is required by the brain to function normally. One quarter of your brain is made from cholesterol so one could say it's the smart fat!

Many people have been brain washed into thinking that dietary cholesterol is unhealthy and dangerous and should be avoided.

Food labels that proudly state that this is a "low fat food" or that this is a "cholesterol free food" only reinforce this fallacy. Thankfully if you do not eat any cholesterol your liver will manufacture all the cholesterol that you need. If you have a healthy liver, the balance of the good cholesterol (HDL) and the bad cholesterol (LDL) and the triglycerides will be favorable in the vast majority of cases. When it comes to keeping your blood fats in the healthy range, it is not so much the avoidance of dietary cholesterol that is important, but the state of your liver that is important.

Thus we can say that a healthy liver is a "fat burning" and a "fat pumping" machine.

Liver Tonics

If you have a sluggish or a fatty liver, a good liver tonic can improve your liver function. These liver tonics help to improve the detoxification and fat burning functions of the liver.

Ingredients in a good liver tonic include:

- St. Mary's Thistle - to repair damaged liver cells
- NAC (N-Acetyl-Cysteine) - to reduce liver damage
- Taurine - to improve bile flow and detoxification
- Selenium - to reduce liver inflammation
- B group vitamins and folinic acid to support the function of liver enzymes. For people with poor ability to detoxify due to fatty liver, the activated form of folic acid, called folinic acid, is preferable to regular folic acid.

You may take all these ingredients individually or combined together in a powerful liver formula such as the LivaTone Plus.

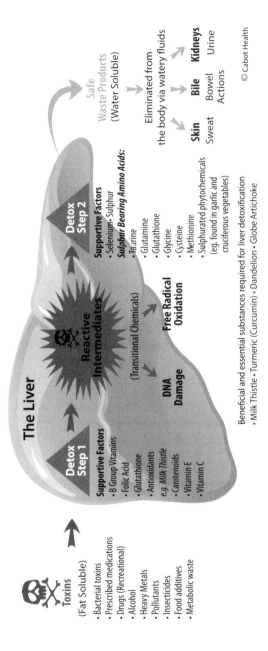

The liver detoxification pathways

Carbohydrates

Carbohydrates are different forms of simple sugars linked together.

Many people do not understand what carbohydrates are. They will often say carbohydrates are confined to cakes, bread, sweets or pasta. Yes it's true that these foods are high in carbohydrates, but fruits and vegetables also contain some carbohydrate. If you were to eat huge amounts of fruit and starchy vegetables every day you would be getting excessive carbohydrate, which would be absorbed as glucose and could be turned into fat. However it is difficult to eat huge amounts of unprocessed carbohydrates because they are high in fiber and take much longer to eat. Conversely, it is very easy to eat huge amounts of refined carbohydrates, as they are low in fiber and are very condensed, so that large amounts of sugar are found in much smaller portion sizes of food.

The most fattening carbohydrate generally comes from plant foods such as cereals, grains, flour and cane sugar. The carbohydrates in fruits, and especially vegetables, are much less fattening than those in grains.

Complex carbohydrates

Complex carbohydrates are much better to eat than simple or refined carbohydrates. Complex carbohydrates do not cause a rapid rise in blood glucose levels, as they are more slowly absorbed than simple carbohydrates. They are absorbed even more slowly if they are eaten with some protein and fat. Because complex carbohydrates take longer to digest, they are more filling and so satisfy the hunger for longer. Be careful when choosing complex carbohydrates, as you do not want breads and pasta made with white flour and sugar and you should choose brown or wild rice over white rice. In other words, choose the unprocessed variety of complex carbohydrates. Food made with white flour and white sugar has had all the fiber and vitamins/minerals removed from it and thus it is of poor nutritional value.

Complex carbohydrates are found in such things as:

- Whole grains - unprocessed
- Whole grain bread
- Legumes - lentils, beans, peas
- Starchy vegetables such as potato, sweet potato, pumpkin, squash, turnips, parsnips, carrots, beetroots and peas etc. These starchy vegetables are higher in carbohydrates than green leafy vegetables. They are also high in fiber, vitamins, minerals and anti-oxidants, and thus can be eaten in moderation.

Green leafy vegetables are very low in carbohydrate and can be eaten freely to fill up on. They are excellent for the liver and bowel, and some of these vegetables, such as green beans and Brussels sprouts can have a beneficial effect on blood glucose and insulin levels. Fill up on generous serves of broccoli, green beans, cabbage, Brussels sprouts, spinach, salad greens, collard greens, and anything green and leafy.

Simple carbohydrates

These are the mono and disaccharides such as glucose, fructose, galactose, sucrose, maltose, and lactose. If the saccharide ends in "ose" it's a simple carbohydrate, the intake of which needs to be controlled. Fructose has a low GI and is the exception. Fructose can be converted into glucose in the liver and intestines; however this is a slow process, which explains why the GI of fructose is only 23.

Simple carbohydrates are found in:

- Pure sugar (glucose)
- Table sugar (sucrose)
- Fructose (found in fruits)
- Maltose (found in beer)
- Lactose (found in cow's milk)

- Honey
- Jam
- Sweets and candies
- Maple syrup
- Corn syrup
- Fruit juices contain fructose and sucrose and in general should be avoided while trying to lose weight. If you are making a fresh vegetable juice for yourself, you may add a small quantity of freshly expressed fruit juice to temper the flavor, but use in moderation. Diabetics should avoid fruit juices.

Fresh fruits are an excellent source of carbohydrates, as they are high in vitamins, minerals and fiber. Although fruit does contain the simple carbohydrate fructose, it does not elevate blood glucose levels as much as other simple carbohydrates. Most calories in fruits come from the simple sugars fructose and sucrose, so you cannot eat unrestricted amounts of fruits.

Canned fruits may be very high in added sugar and the fruit has lost a lot of its nutritional value. Dried fruit is high in sugar and should be avoided if you are overweight; it is best substituted with fresh fruit.

What happens if you eat excess carbohydrate?

After carbohydrate is digested it is absorbed into the blood stream as glucose.

If there is excess glucose in the blood over and above the body's immediate energy needs, the excess glucose will be stored in the form of glycogen. Glycogen is a long chain of glucose molecules linked together.

The body has two storage sites for glycogen – the muscles and the liver cells.

The liver glycogen is most accessible to be broken down into glucose to meet the requirements of the brain for immediate energy. That is why the liver function is so important in keeping blood glucose levels and brain function stable. However the liver's capacity to store glycogen is not unlimited, and can be depleted within 12 hours, if no food is eaten. The capacity of the liver to store glycogen and release it efficiently into the blood stream can be greatly reduced in those with liver problems such as fatty liver, as there are not enough healthy liver cells present to store the required amount of glycogen. In such cases blood glucose levels may fluctuate erratically. If the liver is unable to store excess blood glucose in the form of glycogen, the glucose may be converted into fat, which explains why a dysfunctional liver can lead to weight excess.

If you eat too much carbohydrate, you will exceed the glycogen storage capacity of the liver and muscle cells. In the average person there is around 300 to 400 grams of carbohydrate stored as glycogen in the muscle cells, and 60 to 90 grams in the liver. The liver's stored glycogen is equivalent to around three average sweet energy bars, and is not a lot when you think that this is all there is to keep your brain functioning normally.

Once the capacity of your muscles and liver to store glycogen is full, any excess glucose must be converted into triglyceride fat and is stored as body fat in your adipose tissues. So even though you may be eating fat free carbohydrates, any excess carbohydrate is very easily turned into fat. High carbohydrate fat-free foods can be terribly fattening! **You do not need to eat any fat to become fat!**

Excess dietary carbohydrates send a hormonal signal to your body to store fat in your fatty tissues and also inside your organs. Thus we may develop fatty organs with fat accumulating in the liver, pancreas, spleen, heart and skin. Yes our whole body can become a warehouse for fat simply because the high carbohydrate intake stimulates excessive amounts of the fat storing hormone insulin. High levels of insulin also send signals to your cells not to release any stored fat. This makes it very difficult for your body to use its own stored fat for energy.

What happens when you burn body fat?

When your insulin levels are low your fat cells release free fatty acids, which are a major source of energy for your heart and skeletal muscles. Once you eat carbohydrate your glucose and insulin levels go up, and the insulin suppresses the release of fatty acids from your fat cells. Thus we can say that high levels of insulin stop you burning body fat for energy.

When you burn stored body fat it breaks down into free fatty acids and glycerol, which are then broken down into substances called ketone bodies. This process of fat burning is known as lipolysis and cannot occur without the formation of ketones.

There is nothing bad or dangerous about forming ketones in your body, as ketones are just a sign of using body fat for fuel rather than glucose. The only people who must avoid ketosis are type 1 diabetics, pregnant women or those with liver or kidney failure.

Ketones can be used as fuel by most parts of the body including the heart and brain. Indeed ketones are normal energy sources for many parts of the body.

The lower the dietary carbohydrate intake is, the faster will be the rate of fat burning. By liberating and excreting ketones from your fat stores, you are eliminating the by-products of burning your unwanted fat. This is a very easy way to lose weight because you are eliminating the breakdown products of body fat.

By reducing dietary carbohydrates it is possible to redirect your metabolic pathways into fat burning. This is because you are not consuming enough carbohydrates to equal your energy expenditure and must therefore burn your stored body fat to supply your energy needs. A ketogenic diet is a diet where the dietary carbohydrate intake is so low that the body must burn its fat stores for energy, which leads to the production of ketones in the body.

A ketogenic diet creates a new metabolic pathway for supplying the body with energy by making you a fat burner instead of a carbohydrate burner. For many people this is the most effective and easy initial way to start the weight loss process. See ketogenic diet on page 305.

HIGH LEVELS OF INSULIN NOT ONLY MAKE YOU FATTER, THEY MAKE SURE THAT YOU STAY FAT!

Can gluten make you fat?

We have been taught to think that excess fat and sugar makes us fat, which as far as sugar is concerned is true. But can gluten alone make us overweight or stop us losing weight? You bet it can, I have seen it do this in hundreds of my patients.

Gluten containing foods are naturally high in carbohydrates and many people consume excessive carbohydrates from grains. They would be much better off to get their carbohydrates from vegetables. Other non-gluten containing grains such as rice and corn are also high in carbohydrates – but they are not as fattening as gluten containing grains – very curious!

Why is this?

It is not the calories or the total amount of dietary carbohydrate that is the most important factor, but rather it is the type of molecules in the carbohydrates and how they affect your genes that trigger obesity. If you are gluten intolerant, gluten will turn on your fat genes.

Modern wheat may look like wheat, but it is different from the wheat that was grown hundreds of years ago because–

- It contains a type of gluten that is super-addictive and makes you crave and over eat
- It contains a Super Starch called amylopectin A – this starch is super fattening

The super gluten makes you hungry and potentially addicted to food. In the intestines the proteins in wheat are converted into shorter proteins called "polypeptides" or "exorphins". They are like the endorphins you get from narcotic pain killers. After they attach to the opioid receptors in the brain, you feel euphoric just like a heroin addict. These wheat polypeptides are absorbed from the intestines into the bloodstream and get across the blood brain barrier quickly. They are called "gluteomorphins" after "gluten" and "morphine". Once in the brain they can cause addictive eating behavior and stimulate strong cravings for high carb foods and of course – more gluten!

In summary we can say that wheat is an addictive appetite stimulant!

Another way that gluten makes us fat is that in many people it raises the blood levels of the hormone insulin. Higher insulin levels promote fat storage and hunger.

Modern day wheat is very fattening – such that two slices of whole wheat bread now raise your blood sugar more than two tablespoons of table sugar!

In people with diabetes, both white and whole grain bread raises blood sugar levels 70 to 120 mg/dl over starting levels. Thus the promoted idea that whole wheat grains are healthier than refined wheat grains has been turned on its head

The inflammation caused by gluten saps our energy so we become less inclined to exercise. Have you noticed that after eating a meal high in bread or pasta that you feel tired and slowed down? This is a sign that gluten is not good for you.

It is not just the amount of wheat that we eat but also the hidden components of wheat that drive weight gain and inflammation. Today's wheat is not the wheat eaten by our forebears in the 19th century. It is vastly different so that it has become known as "FrankenWheat" or dwarf wheat. Dwarf wheat has been created via genetic manipulation and hybridization and is a short and stubby type of wheat. Dwarf wheat has much higher amounts of gluten and more chromosomes which code for all sorts of new odd proteins. Thus it brings us into unchartered waters.

Many people try a gluten free diet for a few weeks only, and then seeing no huge improvement, they quit. I can understand this, as gluten foods can be just as addictive as high sugar foods – it is hard to resist and persist!

You need to know that it can take 12 months of a gluten free diet before all the gluten gets out of your body and before the gluten affected cells are fully repaired. This is disappointing, especially if you are a gluten lover. For more information see my book *Gluten, is it making you sick or fat?*

Sources of Gluten in the diet

Gluten is found naturally in the grains wheat, barley, rye and spelt. Some types of oats also contain gluten so it is best to avoid oats. Gluten is an additive in many processed foods.

These gluten containing grains and their flours and other derivative products are found in breads, cereals, crackers, biscuits, muffins, cakes, pizza, pastry, pasta and sauces, unless marked gluten free.

Some gluten-free foods:

Unprocessed poultry, meat, seafood, eggs, dairy products, nuts, seeds and legumes, vegetables and fruits are all gluten free.

Gluten Free	Contain Gluten
Amaranth	Wheat
Buckwheat	Barley
Corn	Rye
Millet	Spelt
Quinoa	Some types of oats
Rice	
Sorghum	
Teff	

Sweeteners

It seems that everyone's taste buds are getting sweeter. A report from the US Department of Agriculture shows a steady increase in the use of sweeteners with an increase from 123 pounds per person in 1980 to 152 pounds annually per person by 1999. Sugar consumption was only 12 pounds per person annually in the early 1800s.

It is normal for almost everyone to desire or even crave very sweet foods at different times during the day. These cravings can become particularly strong if we are highly stressed, our blood glucose is low, or if we have high levels of insulin (hyperinsulinemia). Hormonal imbalances can also make us crave sugar during the pre-menstrual phase of the cycle, after childbirth and during menopause.

The worst type of sugar to eat is refined sugar. Even so called "natural" sugar substitutes such as honey, raw sugar, molasses, barley malt, palm sugar, maple syrup, date sugar, etc. can be unhealthy if eaten in large amounts, as they can elevate blood glucose levels and thus insulin levels. These high insulin levels will hormonally direct the body to turn the sugar into fat.

Refined sugar or table sugar is known as sucrose. It contains 4 calories per gram and has a GI of 65. Sucrose causes a rise in blood glucose and insulin levels, and is best avoided in those with Syndrome X and weight problems.

It is always wise to use the most natural sweeteners available, as the body has enzyme systems that are able to absorb and digest natural foods. Artificial and chemically altered foods are difficult to metabolize and overwork the liver, and may produce harmful chemical waste products in the process. Over many years the safety or harmful effects of artificial and chemically altered sweeteners will become apparent.

Below we take a look at the various sugar substitutes that are available today for those who love the taste of "sweet".

Alternative Sweeteners to table sugar (sucrose)

These sugars are mainly nutritive sugars meaning that they contain calories. They all cause rapid elevations in the blood glucose and insulin levels in those with Syndrome X or diabetes.

- Barley malt
- Honey
- Glucose
- Caramelized sugar
- Brown sugar
- Raw sugar
- Invert sugar (contains glucose and levulose)
- Dextrose
- Maltose
- Molasses
- Maple syrup and maple sugar
- Date sugar
- Evaporated cane juice (sucrose)
- Rice syrup
- Corn syrup
- High fructose corn syrup (contains glucose and fructose)

Fructose (crystalline) is a natural fruit sugar. It is 1.5 to 2 times sweeter than table sugar (sucrose), and thus smaller amounts can be used. Crystalline fructose can be used in cooking and baking and causes the baked product to brown faster. Although fructose contains 4 calories per gram (the same as sucrose), due to its low GI, it does not cause such a large and rapid rise in blood glucose levels as sucrose does.

Sugar alcohols

Sugar alcohols are good for those wanting to lose weight.

Sugar alcohols are derived from sugar molecules but chemically are really alcohols; however they do not have the intoxicating effects of alcohol. Sugar alcohols vary in sweetness from as sweet as sugar to half as sweet as sugar. The better known sugar alcohols are xylitol, mannitol, erythritol, sorbitol and lactitol. Sugar alcohols are also known as polyols and can be used as sugar substitutes by diabetics or those on a low-carbohydrate diet.

Sugar alcohols are incompletely absorbed from the gut and because of this they can produce a laxative effect if overused. Sugar alcohols are not metabolized by the body but they may be included in the total carbohydrate count on food labels. They are often used in sugar free chewing gum or low carbohydrate confectionery.

Stevia

Stevia is a safe non-caloric herbal sweetener.

Stevia is a sweetener extracted from a South American plant called Stevia Rebaudiana and has a very long history of worldwide use.

Stevia herb in its unprocessed form is very sweet, being about 15 times sweeter than table sugar. Stevia extracts in the form of steviosides are hundreds of times sweeter then table sugar, so you only need tiny amounts.

The extraordinary sweetness of Stevia is due to a complex molecule called Stevioside, which is a glycoside that is composed of glucose, sophorose and steviol.

Different forms of Stevia

Stevia comes in different forms - leaves (fresh & dried), liquid, tablets and powder. The taste of Stevia can vary depending upon the brand name, and some brands will have a slight liquorice aftertaste while others will not. Stevia tastes slightly different from sugar and although pleasant in taste, it can be an acquired taste.

Stevia tablets

These can be dissolved in hot beverages like tea and coffee and are convenient to carry around in your purse. The amount can vary from ½ to 2 tablets per cup.

Fresh stevia leaves

If you chew a leaf picked from a stevia plant you will experience a long-lasting very sweet taste that could be compared to liquorice. You may be able to buy some stevia cuttings and plant them in your garden or on the balcony. Stevia grows best outdoors in hot sunny climates. You can use the fresh leaves to sweeten your drinks.

Dried stevia leaves

The dried leaf is a lot sweeter than a fresh leaf. If you add crushed dried leaves to tea or coffee you will need to adjust the amount to suit your palate - use very small amounts to begin with. Many people make the mistake of using too much stevia, and then complain about the flavor.

Dried stevia leaves can be used to sweeten spicy curries, sweet and sour stir-fries and sweet sauces. Generally speaking 2 to 4 dried leaves are required.

Stevia powder - green

The powder is produced by grinding dried leaves and is about 20 times sweeter than sugar. Although it can be added to drinks and hot dishes it has a stronger after taste than other forms of stevia. Generally speaking the white stevia extract powder, stevia tablets or clear liquid stevia are more pleasant with only a slight or negligible after taste.

Stevia powder - white

White stevia extract powder contains 90% of sweet glycosides and is around 300 times sweeter than sugar. It is the most popular form of stevia having the least after taste.

Liquid stevia concentrates

Usually only a few drops are needed to sweeten a cup of tea or coffee, a glass of homemade lemonade or iced tea. They are found in health food stores and come in dropper-type bottles of various sizes.

Safety of Stevia

Stevia can be used as an alternative to artificial sweeteners and sugar in those with weight excess, Syndrome X and type 2 diabetes.

According to research Stevia does not affect blood glucose levels and some studies show that Stevia may reduce blood glucose levels

Stevioside has been used safely among Indians in Paraguay and Brazil for over 200 years and also in Japan for over 30 years. It has been found to be safe and generally free of side effects and so far there have not been any reports of stevia plant toxicity.

Stevia in its pure form, whether it be called Stevia, Stevia extract, Stevioside, or Stevia concentrate, does not adversely affect blood levels of glucose or insulin.

Stevia and Weight Loss

Stevia is an exceptional aid to those trying to lose weight because it has ZERO CALORIES.

One ounce (28grams) of sugar contains 50 calories. One ounce of sugar is approximately 2 teaspoons of sugar and it is not uncommon for an average person to consume 360 grams (13 ounces) of sugar providing 650 calories every day. By replacing the sugar with stevia or Nature Sweet Sugar Substitute you will have a valuable aid to long term weight control.

How to use Natural Sweeteners

Stevia or Nature Sweet Sugar Substitute can be used to completely replace added sugar in our diet. We can also use these sweeteners with sugar, which will enable us to use less sugar, while still retaining the taste of sugar. We can combine them with honey, barley malt, rice syrup, molasses, raw brown sugar or tart tasting fruit juices to reduce the amount of sugar in a recipe and our total consumption of sugar. Nature Sweet Sugar can be used in recipes for baked foods, ice cream, puddings and smoothies. It can be added to freshly squeezed lemon juice or other citrus juices with a delicious result. They are stable at high temperatures and can be used in hot dishes and baked foods. However baked foods made with stevia do not rise as much as those made with Nature Sweet Sugar Substitute. Stevia is not suitable as the sole sweetener in cakes or breads, which require yeast to rise. This is because sugar is needed to stimulate the rising properties of yeast. In such cases use Nature Sweet Sugar Substitute. Artificial sweeteners such as aspartame and saccharin have an obvious after taste and aspartame is unstable when heated.

CONVERSION RATES OF STEVIA		
Amount of sugar or Nature Sweet Sugar Substitute	Equivalent amount of stevia extract powder	Equivalent amount of liquid stevia concentrate
1 teaspoon	a pinch to 1/16 teaspoon	2 to 4 drops or 1 tablet
1 tablespoon	¼ teaspoon	6 to 9 drops or 3 tablets
1 cup	1 teaspoon	1 teaspoon

The above conversions are approximate for the following reasons -

• The sweetness may vary depending upon the brand of stevia used

- Sour or tart foods like lemons, grapefruits, limes, pineapple, green apples or cranberries need more stevia than naturally sweet foods like pears, ripe kiwi fruits or bananas.

Personal taste - some like it sweeter than others

Nature Sweet Sugar Substitute

After extensive research and development, Cabot Health has formulated Nature Sweet Sugar Substitute - a 100% natural granular sugar alternative.

Nature Sweet Sugar Substitute is a mixture of -

- Maltitol is derived from tapioca and has 70-90 % the sweetness of sugar. It is not metabolized by oral bacteria, so it does not promote tooth decay.
- Erythritol is naturally found in fruits and vegetables including grapes, melons and pears and is 60-70% as sweet as table sugar. It is almost non-caloric and does not affect blood sugar and does not cause tooth decay.
- Inulin is a natural polysaccharide. Nature Sweet's inulin comes from chicory root. Inulin promotes growth of good intestinal bacteria (is a prebiotic) and is a form of soluble fibre.
- Stevia comes from a herb and is approximately 300 times sweeter than sugar; it has no effect on blood sugar levels.

Benefits of Nature Sweet Sugar Substitute -

- 100% natural and gluten free
- Ideal for use in weight loss programs
- Not cooling in the mouth like Xylitol
- Perfect for everyone including   diabetics, and children
- Great in tea/coffee
- Easy to use in all your favorite recipes
- No additives
- Does not cause tooth decay

Here is a recipe using Nature Sweet Sugar Substitute

Apricot Flummery

500g	*apricots, halved and stoned*
¼ cup	*Nature Sweet Sugar Substitute*
1 cup	*water*
¾ cup	*chilied evaporated milk (Carnation)*
1 tbspn	*lemon juice*
2 tsp	*powdered gelatine*

Gently simmer apricots, water, Nature Sweet and lemon juice until fruit is tender. Pour off syrup into a bowl. Sprinkle on the gelatine and stir until dissolved. Return syrup to fruit. Adjust sweetness now - more Nature Sweet for extra sweetness or more lemon juice if too sweet. Pour mixture into a bowl and place in fridge to set. When firm, pureè with a stick blender. Meanwhile (using electric beaters) beat chilied evaporated milk until it is light and frothy. Volume should increase by about 3 to 1. Fold milk mixture through fruit mixture until well combined. Pour into bowl and return to fridge to set. Served with icecream. *Serves 6.*

Note: all stone fruits are suitable for this recipe. Simply adjust sweetness.

Artificial chemical sweeteners

- Aspartame
- Neotame
- Saccharin
- Cyclamates
- Sucralose
- Acesulfame - K

The Glycemic Index (GI) of sugars and sweeteners can vary significantly. Many low GI sweeteners are mixed with high GI sweeteners as fillers. This is true if powdered sweeteners are mixed with fillers such as dextrose or maltodextrin. The addition of these high GI fillers can affect the blood glucose levels if multiple packets of the sweetener are used over the day.

High GI sweeteners and sugars are often disguised in foods and appear on the label as such things as glucose polymers, dextrose, maltodextrins or invert sugar.

Saccharin

Saccharin was discovered in 1879 and is a zero-calorie sugar substitute that is approximately 300 times sweeter than sugar. Large amounts of saccharin have been shown to cause cancer in laboratory animals. So far human studies have not shown an increased risk of cancers in saccharin users although the long-term effect of saccharin in humans is still not known.

Sucralose

Sucralose is synthesized by chlorinating the sugar sucrose. Research has found that sucralose can cause health problems in laboratory animals. At this time the long-term safety of sucralose in humans is unknown.

Aspartame

Aspartame was discovered in 1965 and is found in products such as Equal and Nutrasweet. Aspartame is comprised of methanol, phenylalanine and aspartic acid. Methanol is wood alcohol, which breaks down into formaldehyde in the body after ingestion. The FDA and the Dallas based Aspartame Consumer Safety Network have received thousands of consumer complaints about symptoms possibly related to aspartame use. Complaints have included headaches, seizures, depression, blurred vision and numerous neurological disorders. Dr Nuri Farber and Dr John Olney from the Washington University Medical School in St. Louis, Missouri believe aspartame is a suspicious causative factor in various health problems. The November 1996 edition of the Journal of Neuropathology and Experimental Neurology, contains their statement that "In the past two decades, brain tumor rates have risen in several industrialized countries, including the USA. Compared to other environmental factors putatively linked to brain tumors, the artificial sweetener aspartame is a promising candidate to explain the recent increase in incidence and degree of malignancy of brain tumors. Evidence potentially implicating aspartame includes an early animal study revealing a exceedingly high incidence of brain tumors in aspartame - fed rats, compared to no brain tumors in concurrent controls. We conclude that there is need for reassessing the carcinogenic potential of aspartame". (Olney, Farber, 1996). The FDA issued a statement in 1996 that "A recently published medical journal article raises the question whether any increased incidence in the number of persons with brain tumors in the USA is associated with the marketing of aspartame. Analysis of the National Cancer Institute's public database on cancer incidence in the USA does not support an association between the use of aspartame and the increased incidence of brain tumors. The FDA stands behind its original approval decision, but the agency remains ready to act if credible scientific evidence is presented to it." Despite this assurance from the FDA there are many researchers who do not agree with the FDA.

> **For more information visit** - www.dorway.com You can also E-mail Betty Martini at Mission-Possible-USA@altavista.net from this site.

Betty is an activist who believes that aspartame should be banned and she can recommend several authoritative books on this subject. At this present time I believe that it is wise to avoid the artificial chemical aspartame as a sweetener, or foods which contain it.

The proponents of aspartame will tell you that it does not cause tooth decay and can help with weight control, however the natural sweeteners such as sugar alcohols and stevia also have these advantages.

Acesulfame

This artificial sweetener was approved by the FDA in 1988 and is a derivative of aceoacetic acid. This is a synthetic chemical, which is probably not metabolized by the body and is 200 times sweeter than sugar. The likelihood of long term danger in humans from this artificial chemical is currently unknown.

The long-term use of all the artificial chemical sweeteners has not been proven to be completely safe. I believe that substituting stevia or sugar alcohols for aspartame, acesulfame and saccharin is a safer alternative for those who wish to avoid sugar.

Dietary Fats - The good, the bad and the ugly

Most people struggling to lose weight try to avoid dietary fats and often meticulously scour food labels to determine the fat content of foods. Fat has become a dirty word, probably because it is a very calorie dense food providing 9 calories per gram of fat.

We know that it is not just the amount of calories that you consume that makes you fat - it is more important to choose the source of the calories wisely. Dietary fat is good for you, and a blanket ban on all dietary fat means that we throw out the good fats along with the bad fats.

Dietary fat does not cause blood insulin levels to rise significantly, so you do not have such high amounts of the fat producing hormone insulin in your body.

In people who eat no fat, there can be health problems, as fat is an essential dietary item. Without any dietary fat your metabolic rate will slow down so that you burn calories less efficiently. This is because the cells and their tiny internal organs are made of essential fatty acids. If you do not get enough dietary essential fats, your cells will suffer, and their membranes will be of inferior structural quality. The cells will not function efficiently and will not produce enough cellular energy, resulting in a sluggish metabolism. Essential fatty acids and cholesterol make your cell membrane walls flexible, so that nutritional substances are able to take fat out of the cell. Californian endocrinologist Dr Diana Schwarzbein has been researching dietary fat intake for more than 20 years. She has found that low fat diets are always followed by a decline in health. Indeed her research of hundreds of women found that low-fat fanatics eventually increase body fat and may have increased blood pressure.

Your body cannot manufacture its own essential fats, and that is why we say they are essential to obtain from your diet.

Many people on a low fat diet become yo-yo dieters, and as they lose weight their metabolism slows down. When they come off the low fat diet and start to eat "normally" again, their slow metabolism cannot cope with the increased calories; thus they quickly regain the extra pounds, and often more.

We now know that the low-fat message given to us since the 1970s was too simplistic. We know that low fat diets do not work - just look at Australia and the USA, where people have easy access to processed no-fat or low-fat foods, and yet there is an epidemic of obesity and diabetes!

Dietary Fat is Healthy!

Sex hormones, vitamin D, bile and many of the body's natural steroid hormones are made from cholesterol.

Cholesterol is also used to make cell membranes and the insulating sheaths around nerve fibers. Your brain is largely composed of fat – essential fatty acids and cholesterol.

If you do not eat any cholesterol, your liver will make enough cholesterol for your body to survive and use.

Cholesterol is essential in the body for good health.

In my eating program you will get healthy amounts of cholesterol in your diet.

In the past, people have been wrongly educated to avoid foods containing cholesterol (such as eggs, cheese and shellfish), for fear that these foods may raise blood cholesterol levels. We now know that cholesterol is essential in the human body, and that a healthy liver can adjust its production of cholesterol to compensate for increased dietary consumption of cholesterol. If your liver is healthy it will manufacture the good cholesterol called HDL cholesterol, which prevents atherosclerosis. If your liver is unhealthy and fatty, it will manufacture excessive amounts of the bad LDL cholesterol, even if you follow a low fat diet.

Many people who have cholesterol levels above the so called normal range do not eat large amounts of saturated fat and their problem comes from eating too much refined carbohydrate and sluggish liver function.

In a small percentage of the population there exists an inherited defect called "familial hypercholesterolemia", which results in grossly elevated cholesterol levels. In these people there is a genetic impairment of the liver's ability to regulate cholesterol production, and it is necessary to reduce cholesterol containing foods and take cholesterol-lowering medication.

So the good news is that the vast majority of people can eat and enjoy a moderate amount of fatty foods which contain natural fats such as cholesterol

Fats are needed for the healthy appearance of the hair and skin, so those on very low fat diets often look drawn, with a dried out look and dull dry hair.

The metabolic effect in the body of the food you eat is just as important as the calories it contains. So eating fat is OK, as long as you abide by some simple rules -

You cannot eat unlimited amounts of fat, as it is high in calories.

You should choose the good fats and avoid the bad fats, as the latter will slow down your metabolism and increase the risk of a fatty liver.

Understanding dietary fats

Saturated Fats

Butter, lard, animal fats, and some plant fats such as palm oil and coconut oil.

Saturated fats are usually solid at room temperature.

Animal fats are saturated and contain cholesterol, whereas plant fats do not contain any cholesterol.

Unsaturated Fats

Seed and vegetable oils like olive oil, canola oil, and flaxseed oil. Corn oil and safflower oil are very high in polyunsaturated fats, whilst olive oil, avocado and nut oils are high in mono-unsaturated fats.

Unsaturated fats are liquid at room temperature.

The conventional dietary philosophy of today tells us to minimize cholesterol. Instead we are told to eat a lot of polyunsaturated fat. Many people follow this theory and use loads of margarine and cheap processed polyunsaturated oils; but we still have a very high incidence of diabetes and obesity in our fat conscious society. A presentation by Dr Tirshwell at the 1999 AHA Conference reported the findings of a study, which looked at the cholesterol levels of stroke victims compared to cholesterol levels amongst healthy subjects. Surprisingly it showed that brain hemorrhages were significantly more common in subjects with low cholesterol. *(REF. 27)*

You see it's not as simple as avoiding saturated fats and replacing them with polyunsaturated fats - it's the quality of the fats that we eat that is so important. We need to avoid processed hydrogenated fats, deep fried foods, and fats that are oxidized (not fresh).

We do not need a low fat diet; we need the right fat diet!

Essential Fatty Acids

Essential fatty acids (EFAs) are essential to get in the diet and are essential for good health. Because our food has become increasingly processed and many people erroneously follow low fat diets, I have found that deficiencies of essential fatty acids are very common. Your liver can manufacture cholesterol, but it cannot manufacture the essential fatty acids (EFAs).

Sources of omega 3 EFAs are -

- Egg yolks, especially from hens that are fed vegetables
- Nuts, especially walnuts and walnut oil (great on salad dressing)
- Seeds - flaxseeds, chia and hemp
- Cold water fish such as mackerel, trout, cod, herring, tuna, salmon and sardines
- Grass fed lamb and beef
- Fish oil
- Canola oil – this is generally highly processed and genetically modified and I do not recommend it
- The leaves and seeds of most plants

Sources of omega 6 EFAs are -

- Evening primrose oil
- Borage seed oil (starflower oil)
- Blackcurrant seed oil
- Egg yolks
- Dark green leafy vegetables
- Seeds
- Whole grains

Sources of omega 9 fatty acids are -

- Olives and olive oil
- Avocados and avocado oil
- Nut oils including peanut oil
- Sesame oil
- Hemp seeds

Omega 9 fatty acids are not essential in the diet, but still they have great advantages for an efficient metabolism.

Increase the essential fatty acids in your diet

Many people believe that they get enough EFAs by consuming cooking oils, which are relatively cheap and are available in plastic containers on super market shelves. These commercial oils have been processed with chemicals at high temperatures; this damages their original essential fatty acids.

I strongly encourage you to buy only the good quality, cold pressed, unrefined oils that are usually available in glass containers. The oils are better preserved if the glass container is dark colored as it keeps the light out. Essential fatty acids are very fragile and are easily damaged by exposure to heat, air and light. Keep your oils in a cool dark cupboard.

Olive, coconut or palm oils are best for high temperature cooking such as stir fries or sautéing. Do not cook with flaxseed oil, or indeed heat it in any way, as you will damage and oxidize its fragile EFAs.

Healthy ways to increase your EFAs

Nuts - such as walnuts, pecans, Brazil, almonds, macadamias, hazelnuts and cashews. When it comes to peanut butters buy only the natural types, as many commercial smooth peanut butters are adulterated with large amounts of trans-fatty acids.

Salad dressings – these are a good way of increasing your intake of beneficial EFAs. Mayonnaise, cold pressed oils, such as olive oil, flaxseed oil, hemp seed oil, nut oils and avocado oil. Combine these oils with lemon juice or apple cider vinegar for slimming healthy salad dressings. Flaxseed oil is nice to add to your salads or dry baked vegetables, as it has a very mild taste. Do not use the cheap, processed and polyunsaturated cooking oils for salad dressings. Replace them with unrefined cold pressed virgin olive oil, seed oils, avocado oil or nut oils. We need to eat a lot of salads to keep our liver healthy, so the salad dressings will be a regular source of EFAs in our diet. Many fat - free salad dressings are unhealthy, being loaded with sugar and chemicals and do not taste that great - indeed they are bad enough to put you off eating salads!

Spreads - tahini, humus, nut spreads (unprocessed), avocados and olive oil.

Start to eat fish regularly, especially the cold water varieties of fish and/or take a fish oil supplement.

Eggs are an excellent source of EFAs as well as a complete protein – choose free range.

Eat plenty of dark green leafy vegetables and some eggplant to increase the healthful EFAs.

Eat avocados regularly as they are high in EFAs and vitamin E and help to eradicate cellulite.

In general the average person consumes too much omega 6 fatty acids compared to omega 3 fatty acids. This is because we consume excess amounts of cheap processed refined oils made from soy, canola, safflower and corn, which are very high in omega 6 EFAs and relatively deficient in omega 3 EFAs.

We do not eat sufficient amounts of foods high in the omega 3 EFAs such as fish, nuts, nut oils, seeds and egg yolks. This imbalance of omega 6 to omega 3 EFAs, combined with the over consumption of trans-fatty acids found in margarine and many snack foods, partially explains why in this day and age we have such high levels of obesity, heart disease and inflammatory diseases and dementia.

Trans-fatty acids - the really bad fats!

Trans-fatty acids are one of the worst public health disasters in history! Trans-fatty acids cause insulin resistance, slow metabolism, and increase the risk of diabetes, heart disease and blindness; they are widely used in processed and packaged foods.

Trans-fatty acids are man made processed fats that originate from vegetable oils and margarine is the best known example. Trans-fatty acids are manufactured by taking a vegetable oil, and forcing additional hydrogen atoms into the carbon chains in the oil. That's why these oils are called partially hydrogenated oils. This hydrogenation process makes the fat more saturated, which means it becomes solid, albeit a soft solid, at room temperature. Thus it is easy to spread and is convenient.

Trans-fatty acids and other partially hydrogenated vegetable oils are totally unnatural - we could even say they are alien to the body, as our cells find it very hard to use them. The liver does not know how to utilize trans-fatty acids efficiently either and they may accumulate in the liver causing a fatty liver.

Trans-fatty acids also cause your body to secrete more insulin which is another reason they cause weight gain. Please replace trans-fats with naturally occurring saturated and mono-unsaturated oil, including butter, coconut oil and olive oil.

Sources of the Trans-fatty acids

- Most types of margarine are high in trans-fatty acids.
- Foods deep-fried in polyunsaturated vegetable oils such as chips and batter. When you deep-fry any foods in sunflower, canola, corn and other vegetable oils, you will cause the production of unhealthy trans-fatty acids. It is healthier and less fattening to fry foods in saturated fats such as butter, ghee, palm or coconut oil, which are more stable and not as easily damaged by extreme high temperatures.
- Potato chips in packets - they may state they are cholesterol free, but so what? Cholesterol is not the enemy!
- Many fast foods and takeaway foods.

- Many pastries and packaged foods - biscuits, cookies, cakes, buns, breads, commercially baked goods, doughnuts and muffins, etc. If a product label says it contains vegetable oils there is a 90% chance it is cheap hydrogenated oil.

- Many processed foods such as some brands of mayonnaise, salad dressings containing cheap vegetable oils, some brands of peanut butter, dips and spreads, etc.

- Many brands of candy bars and snack bars.

Your Body Type

There are four classic body shapes or body types; they are the –

- Android Body Type – apple shape
- Gynaeoid Body Type – pear shape
- Thyroid Body Type – long, skinny and bony shape
- Lymphatic Body Type – round and puffy all over shape

The different body types are classified according to the anatomical proportions of their bones and where they store fat.

Each body type has unique hormonal and metabolic characteristics, which explains why some body types gain weight easily and are more prone to cellulite. Your body type also determines the areas of your body where excess fat will accumulate.

The vast majority of people will belong to one of these four body types. Around 10% of people are a combination of two body types. The body types are genetically determined so you will probably find someone in your own family with the same body type as yourself. Your body type determines your metabolic type and is important to know because it explains the foods that may cause problems for you. When you avoid the foods that are incompatible with your body type, weight loss becomes much easier.

Android Body Type

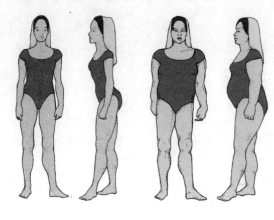

Android ideal   *Android overweight*

Approximately 40% of women and the vast majority of men belong to this body type. It is characterized by broad shoulders, strong muscular arms and legs, a narrow pelvis and narrow hips. The waistline does not curve inwards very much, so the trunk has a somewhat straight up and down appearance. Android women have a boyish figure, and are usually good at sports and are athletic and strong.

Android-shaped people have an anabolic metabolism, which leads to a body building tendency in the upper part of the body. Weight gain occurs in the upper part of the body and on the front of the abdomen, so that an apple-shape may develop.

Android Body Type Weight Control Tablets contain the herbs Red Clover, Dong Quai and Milk Thistle and the liver nutrients choline and inositol and the fiber chitosan.

Gynaeoid Body Type

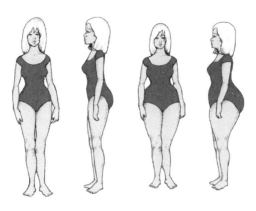

Gynaeoid ideal   *Gynaeoid overweight*

Approximately 40% of women belong to this body type, which is characterized by small to medium shoulders, a narrow tapering waistline and wide hips. Weight gain tends to occur on the buttocks and thighs, which accentuates the pear shape of the Gynaeoid type. The hips and thighs curve outwards and excess weight gain occurs below the waistline. Gynaeoid women are "estrogen dominant", which means that the hormone estrogen has the greatest influence in their body shape. They often have a relative deficiency of the other female hormone called progesterone. Excessive estrogen promotes fat deposition and cellulite around the hips, thighs and buttocks. Natural progesterone balances the effect of estrogen and helps to reduce weight from the hips and thighs.

The Gynaeoid body type is uncommon in men, however very occasionally you will find a man who falls into this category.

Gynaeoid Body Type Weight Control Tablets contain the herbs Wild Yam, Parsley Piert, Vitex Agnes Castus, Gymnema Sylvestre and chromium picolinate to assist their weight loss.

Thyroid Body Type

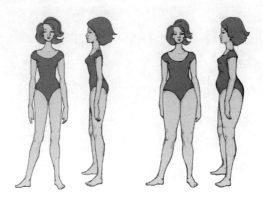

Thyroid ideal   *Thyroid overweight*

Approximately 10% of women and 5% of men belong to this body type, which is characterized by a fine (small) bone structure, relatively long limbs compared to the trunk and a long narrow neck. Thyroid shaped people often become dancers or fashion models, and can be described as having a 'race-horse' or 'greyhound' appearance.

Thyroid types have a high metabolic rate and do not have as many fat cells as the other body types, which means that they do not gain weight easily; thus they can often eat much larger amounts than their friends without showing the effects. We call them thyroid types because they have such a rapid and efficient metabolism, and not because they are more likely to suffer with thyroid diseases.

Interestingly thyroid women are often naughty with their diet, in that they miss meals and live on stimulants, such as caffeine, diet sodas, fizzy soft drinks, sugar and cigarettes.

Blood sugar imbalances often result from the overuse of stimulants, which may lead to fatigue, but thyroid types try to overcome this with more stimulants!

They do not put on weight easily because they do not build

muscle easily and they do not store fat. They have a smaller number of fat cells than the other body types so there are not many places on their body where they can store fat. They often try to put on weight as they feel too skinny. If they become very underweight, especially in combination with smoking and a deficiency of nutrients, their estrogen levels may become very low. Low estrogen levels lead to a reversible loss of breast tissue and feminine curves, and in the long term osteoporosis.

Thyroid Body Type Weight Control Tablets contain the minerals chromium picolinate, magnesium and zinc combined with glutamine, vitamin B 5 and the herbs Liquorice and Ginseng to balance their metabolism.

Lymphatic Body Type

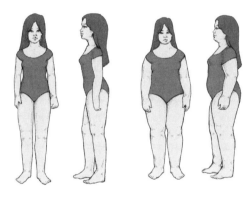

Lymphatic ideal   *Lymphatic overweight*

Approximately 10% of women and 5% of men belong to this body type, which is characterized by weight gain all over the body.

The limbs have a thick puffy or spongy appearance and the bone structure is not very visible. There is a layer of fat and fluid all over the body, which may be excessively thick. These people have often been plagued with weight excess since childhood. Lymphatic people have a very slow metabolic rate, which causes them to gain weight very easily. They also have an inefficient lymphatic system, which leads to fluid retention and makes lymphatic people appear fatter than they really are. Cellulite is common in this body type, with deposits of fat swollen with lymphatic fluid, giving a dimpled appearance on thick puffy limbs.

Lymphatic types may have imbalances in pituitary hormones, such as prolactin and growth hormone mediators, and overall they are hypersensitive to hormones.

Lymphatic Body Type Weight Control Tablets contain the herbs Fenugreek, Celery, Horseradish and Fennel combined with kelp, cayenne, rutin, selenium and vitamin B 6 to assist with weight loss.

For information on your Body Type and the Body Type Weight Control Tablets phone 623 334 3232 in the USA or 02 4655 8855 in Australia and speak to a nutritionist.

> *To discover your Body Type visit https://www.liverdoctor.com/ body-type-questionnaire/ and do the interactive questionnaire on line – get your answer now!*

The Apple Shape versus the Pear Shape

Apple shaped people accumulate excess weight in the trunk and inside the abdominal cavity and on the abdominal wall.

People who carry excess fat around the abdomen are at an increased risk of diabetes and heart disease. These people are commonly Android or Lymphatic Body Types and are more resistant to insulin than those who store most of their body fat in the hips and thighs. The latter are known as pear shaped or Gynaeoid Body Types. According to Dr Cynthia Sites from the Vermont College of Medicine, "efforts to reduce either subcutaneous abdominal fat or intra-abdominal fat should be helpful in reducing the risk of type 2 diabetes in post menopausal women". Their study found that the higher the abdominal fat stores were, the less the body was able to respond to insulin.

How do you know if you are apple shaped?

Measure your waist and hips with a tape measure while unclothed. To do this measure your waist one inch (2.5cms) above the navel, or at its narrowest part, while standing with the abdominal muscles relaxed. If there is no smallest area around the waist, take the measurement at the level of the navel. Then measure your hips at their widest point while standing.

Divide your waist measurement by your hip measurement to get your waist to hip ratio.

A waist to hip ratio of over 0.8 for women, and over 1.0 for men is suggestive of an unfavorable accumulation of fat around the middle, which increases diabetes and heart disease risk.

Can your genes make you fat?

Hunger is one of the biggest reasons why some people cannot stick to a weight loss diet. New research has identified a hunger gene that may be responsible for excessive hunger in some individuals.

It is certainly true that some people experience a lot more hunger than others. Some people adore food and they spend a large part of their waking moments thinking about and planning their next meal. We call them "foodies"!

Other people aren't fussed with food at all, and sometimes forget to eat if they are very engrossed in an activity, or they prefer coffee and cigarettes or alcohol – naughty! The types who crave stimulants instead of food, are usually the Thyroid Body Types.

Personally I don't understand how anyone can forget to eat! Eating is a very pleasurable activity and it provides your body with the nutrients it needs for health, a good mood and physical energy. Unfortunately some people experience a real battle with hunger. Just one week on a weight loss regime is enough to see them pulling their hair out in desperation; wildly craving their favorite comfort foods.

Science can offer a few explanations for this type of experience. Recently a hunger gene called MC4R has been discovered. It seems that some people inherit a defective copy of this gene from their parents and this predisposes them to ravenous hunger for their entire life. You only need to inherit the gene from one of your parents to be affected. Bummer at least it could have been a recessive gene! People with the defective hunger gene spend most of their life overweight; they generally start gaining excess weight in childhood.

This research is still in its infancy and you cannot go to your local pathology company and be tested for this fat gene yet.

What can you do if you have inherited this fat gene from a parent?

Does it mean you are destined to spend your entire life overweight and hungry?

Thankfully NO - the strategies in this book can help!

You have probably noticed that lately, a new gene that codes for a specific disease or imbalance is discovered nearly every month. We now know there are diabetes genes, obesity genes, breast cancer genes, Alzheimer's genes and so on. However, having a gene for a particular disease does not mean you are doomed! Your genes are not always your destiny. There was a brilliant article published in Time Magazine called *Why your DNA is not your Destiny*. You can read the article at http://www.time.com/time/magazine/article/0,9171,1952313-1,00.html This article explains the concept of epigenetics. Basically this means that several factors in our environment affect the way our genes behave. Genes can be turned on or turned off. You may have a gene for a particular disease, but the gene may be kept silenced (or turned off) for your entire life. What you eat, what you think and the way you live all determine whether the gene will become activated or not. A gene symbolizes potential, not destiny. For example not every woman with breast cancer genes will develop breast cancer; these women have a 40 to 80 percent increased risk. If they smoke, drink excess alcohol, are deficient in vitamin D, selenium or iodine, or are overweight, their risk is much higher.

Natural ways to keep the hunger gene switched off or down regulated

- Limit your intake of sugar and high carbohydrate foods like flour, pasta, gluten, white potatoes and breakfast cereals. Eating these foods triggers your pancreas to release the hormone insulin. Too much insulin is a bad thing because it promotes fat storage and fluid retention, but insulin also makes you hungry. People with high insulin levels become very ravenous and they have strong cravings for carbohydrate rich foods. Thankfully there are herbs and nutrients that support the function of insulin – thus your pancreas needs to make less insulin. These include the herbs Gymnema and Bitter melon, and the nutrients chromium, lipoic acid and magnesium. They are all found in Glicemic Balance capsules. Taking one capsule with each meal or at least one capsule twice daily, can help reduce your appetite and make sticking to a diet so much easier.

- If you get hungry, but do not need to eat, try Synd-X Slimming Protein Powder mixed with unsweetened milk in a blender. Synd-X powder contains extremely high protein and virtually no carbohydrates and also extra taurine and glutamine to help metabolism in the liver. It tastes sweet because it is flavored with stevia.

- Eat plenty of protein and good fats. Eating protein at each meal is a great way to keep you full and satisfied for hours. Protein helps to keep your blood sugar stable and prevents dips in blood sugar that leave you in search of the cookie jar. Protein powder smoothies are a convenient, delicious and healthy way of boosting your protein intake. Synd-X Slimming Protein powder is made of whey protein and contains no artificial ingredients at all. It is naturally sweetened with the herb stevia. Including some good fats in your diet will also help to keep you full and satisfied for longer. Dressing a salad with oil such as olive, macadamia or coconut oil will make it more palatable and also help you absorb more antioxidants from the vegetables.

- Drink plenty of water. Often when you feel hungry, it is really water that your body is craving. Having a glass of water or a cup of tea is a great way to stave off hunger between meals. Don't drink diet soda because the sweet taste will actually make you hungrier in the long run.

- Try to keep calm. Cool, calm and collected people rarely binge eat. Stress is one of the biggest factors that take people off the rails when it comes to their diet. Many people use eating as a coping mechanism to deal with difficulties in their life and unpleasant emotions such as loneliness, guilt, grief, fear, frustration or anger. Seeing a counselor or clinical hypnotherapist regularly, can help to overcome the emotional imbalance that leads to overeating.

- Magnesium supplements can be most beneficial. Magnesium helps to physically relax your nervous system and muscles. This helps to make you calmer during the day and improves your quality of sleep at night.

No matter what genes you've been dealt, it is possible to reduce excessive hunger and stick with a healthy diet. Keep your appetite under control and feel the mental benefits.

Hormonal Imbalances and Weight Gain

Are hormonal imbalances making you fat?

Years ago doctors, family members and friends would often advise women who battled with a weight problem that it was due to hormonal problems or their glands. In the early 20th century there was very little understanding about the ways that hormones affected the body. No real help was available and the patient just accepted that this was the way she/he had to remain. Today things have improved greatly and we now know that specific hormones can affect metabolism and hunger and also the areas where excessive fat will be deposited. We are able to measure accurately the blood levels of all the body's hormones, and can pin point the significant hormonal imbalances that will trigger weight gain.

Thyroid Gland Dysfunction

Dysfunction of the thyroid gland can have a profound effect on the metabolism and therefore weight. An overactive thyroid gland produces excess amounts of thyroid hormone, which usually results in weight loss even though there is a

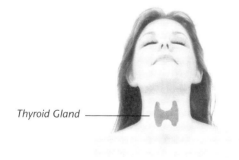

Thyroid Gland

voracious appetite. Conversely, an under active thyroid gland does not produce adequate amounts of thyroid hormone and the metabolism slows down. Even a slightly underactive thyroid gland can make it much harder to lose weight.

The symptoms of an underactive thyroid gland can include-

Easy weight gain, fluid retention, constipation, low body temperature, hair loss, dryness of the skin and a general slowing of bodily and mental functions. The condition of an underactive thyroid gland is called hypothyroidism, while the condition of an over active thyroid gland is called hyperthyroidism. Hypothyroidism is very common, especially in women. It is associated with fatigue and muscle weakness, so there is not much inclination to exercise, which leads to more weight gain.

The function of the thyroid gland can be easily checked with a simple blood test, which measures the level of the thyroid hormones. The thyroid gland produces the hormone called thyroxine, which is also known as T4. Most of the thyroxine (T4) is converted in the body into a more active form of thyroid hormone called triiodothyronine (T3). T3 has a much greater ability to stimulate the energy factories (mitochondria) inside the body's cells. T3 tells your cells to burn food calories at a faster rate and so it is essential to produce enough T 3 in your body.

Sometimes the body does not produce the right shape of T 3 and instead produces an abnormally shaped form of T 3 called Reverse T 3 (R T 3). This Reverse shape of T 3 does not work and if produced in excess amounts can block weight loss. If there is sluggish liver function, or fatty liver, or gluten intolerance, this can produce excess amounts of the useless R T 3. It is possible to measure the amount of T 3 and Reverse T 3 with a simple blood test. In people with abnormally high R T 3 levels supplements of selenium are indicated.

Blood tests for thyroid gland function

The blood tests for thyroid gland function should ideally measure the following -

Hormone	Normal Range
Thyroid Stimulating Hormone (TSH). TSH stimulates the thyroid gland to make more thyroid hormone.	0.5 to 2.5 mU/L – this is ideal. However many labs will report the normal range as up to 5, which is way too high (underactive thyroid)
Free T 4	9.0 to 24.0 pmol/L
Free T 3	2.2 to 5.4 pmol/L
Reverse T3	140-500 pmol/L
Urinary iodine concentration	Over 100mcg per litre
Thyroid antibodies *Anti-thyroglobulin Antibody (TgAb)*	Cut off titre = <100
Anti-microsomal Antibody Ab (TPOAb)*	Cut off titre = <100
*This antibody is also called thyroid peroxidase	

If the TSH is found to be above the normal range, this means that the thyroid gland is under active. For ideal metabolism you want your TSH to be less than 2.6mU/L.

Note: Low thyroid function is often a missed diagnosis. This is because the reference range for TSH in several countries has been changed to 0.2-2.5 mIU/L. This means that many people, who previously have been told that their thyroid function is normal, can now be classified as officially hypothyroid. Unfortunately many labs still report the normal level of TSH as up to 5 mU/L and people who need treatment do not receive it – they can never lose weight.

Ask your doctor for a copy of your blood tests.

If the thyroid gland is only slightly under active (TSH over 3mU/L), we are often able to stimulate it back to normal function by the following -

Improving the diet and avoiding gluten containing foods, which are wheat, rye, barley and oats.

Taking supplemental selenium 100mcg, zinc 5mg, iodine 162mcg and vitamin D 1,000 units daily; these are all combined together in the correct dosage in *Thyroid Health Capsules.* Deficiencies of iodine and selenium are very common and can cause sluggish thyroid function and weight gain.

If the thyroid gland function remains abnormally low after 4 months of nutritional supplementation and a gluten free diet, it will be necessary to take thyroid hormone replacement. This is usually given in the form of tablets containing thyroxine (T 4) – common brands of thyroxine include Synthroid, Eutrosig and Oroxine. Many people worry that taking thyroxine tablets is the same as taking artificial drugs, however this is not correct, as thyroxine tablets are merely replacing a natural hormone that the thyroid gland can, no longer produce by itself. If the dosage is carefully controlled, there are generally no side effects. Often only small doses are required.

In most people the thyroxine tablets work very well and increase the metabolic rate back to normal, so that weight loss occurs and energy levels are restored.

In some people the thyroxine tablets have a good initial response, but become increasingly ineffective over time. This condition is called **thyroid resistance**, and means that the body cells have become resistant to the effect of the hormone thyroxine (T4). In some patients the body is not able to convert the thyroxine (T4) into the more active form of triiodothyronine (T3), so the metabolism slows down. To treat thyroid resistance we can use supplemental selenium and zinc to help the conversion of T4 into T3. This will work in many cases of thyroid resistance; however in very resistant cases it will be necessary to give triiodothyronine (T3) tablets. T3 tablets are available in various brand names such as Cytomel and Tertoxin. In most cases of thyroid resistance we need to give both T4 and T3 tablets to restore normal thyroid hormone balance and metabolism. Typical doses of thyroid hormone are T4, 50 to 100mcg daily and T3, 10 to 20mcg twice daily. You can take T4 and T3 tablets separately or combined together by a compounding chemist. You will need a prescription for these medications and will need to be monitored by your doctor.

In people with thyroid resistance, the addition of T3 tablets can be dramatically effective and enable the patient to lose weight much more easily. Such patients are extremely grateful.

Thyroid replacement made from desiccated pig's thyroid glands is sometimes used today in people who are thyroid resistant and do not respond to T 4 alone. Porcine thyroid extract was the only type of thyroid treatment available during the early 20th century; porcine thyroid is still popular today. Doses of porcine thyroid vary from 20 to 200mg daily, as some people only need a small amount. Porcine thyroid is made by a compounding chemist and is put into capsules.

Thyroid hormone cream, which contains porcine thyroid extract, can be massaged into the skin. This is helpful for those with mild thyroid dysfunction or those who are intolerant to thyroid tablets - see www.liverdoctor.com

Your Basal Body Temperature reflects your Thyroid Function

The basal body temperature is the lowest temperature attained by the body during sleep. It is measured immediately after awakening and before any physical activity has occurred.

In people with an underactive thyroid gland the body temperature falls below normal because of slower metabolism. An overactive thyroid elevates body temperature producing a low grade fever.

The metabolism in your whole body is completely dependent on enzyme function. Importantly enzyme function is highly dependent on body temperature.

If your basal body temperature is below normal, then all the enzymes in every cell of your body will be working too slowly, which means your metabolism will be way too low.

Measuring your basal body temperature (BBT) can pin point a thyroid problem even if your blood tests for thyroid function are seemingly "normal."

This BBT is performed first thing in the morning, upon awakening, and before you become physically active. Tracking basal body temperature over 14 mornings gives you a better average.

Most digital basal thermometers on the market are not accurate enough for this type of thyroid testing, where we are measuring your BBT. A digital thermometer, and also an infrared thermometer, will under read a person's body temperature.

The most accurate thermometer is the old-fashioned mercury thermometer, around which this specific BBT test was originally created and standardized. Mercury thermometers can still be found in many pharmacies. You can also ask for a mercury-based fertility thermometer.

Modern digital-style thermometers are calibrated differently from the mercury type, hence will give inaccurate readings for the BBT test. Only use *the old-fashioned mercury thermometer.*

Technique to test the Basal Body Temperature

Your mercury thermometer should be re-set by shaking it down the night *before* the first morning test, as well as after you have recorded each morning's result. This ensures the thermometer is ready to use well before the next testing. It can take quite a bit of shaking to get the mercury column to go down to below the 35 degrees Celsius (95.0 degrees Fahrenheit) figure on this type of thermometer. You must take your temperature immediately after awakening as any physical activity will increase your temperature, thus preventing you getting the required *basal* reading.

As soon as you wake up, take your temperature, *under the arm in the armpit*, (not under the tongue) for a full 10 minutes. It is vital to place the mercury thermometer underarm, and not under the tongue. Do not move or get out of bed before taking your temperature. Any such activity will raise your basal body temperature, and make the test useless.

It's important to accurately record the readings, as well as try to have those readings taken at about the same time each morning.

For premenopausal women it is important to only measure the temperature on the 2nd, 3rd and 4th morning of their menstrual bleeding.

For men and post menopausal women, the temperature can be taken on any 14 – or more consecutive mornings.

Once you have recorded the 14 readings, work out the average temperature.

Understanding your Basal Body Temperature Results

A healthy human's normal body temperature is considered to be 37 degrees Celsius (98.6 Fahrenheit).

If your average basal body temperature (BBT) reading is *below* 36.5 degrees Celsius (97.7 degrees Fahrenheit), then this is an indication, that you have an underactive thyroid.

The more your average BBT is below 36.5 degrees Celsius (97.7 degrees Fahrenheit), the more your thyroid is underactive. Any average temperature below 36.0 degrees Celsius, (96.8 degrees Fahrenheit) would suggest that your thyroid is starting to become underactive.

In such cases, a TSH reading (done on a blood sample) is also more likely to come back as 2.0mU/L or higher.

Celsius and Fahrenheit Conversions

(°C x 9/5) + 32 = °F   (°F - 32) x 5/9 = °C

For example:

Converting 36.5 degrees Celsius to Fahrenheit:

36.5 x 9 = 328.5

328 divided by 5 = 65.7

65.7 + 32 = 97.7

Sluggish thyroid function is a common hidden problem that prevents many people from being successful with their weight loss programs. For more information see my book Your Thyroid problems Solved.

The Hunger Hormones – Leptin and Ghrelin

Our bodies manufacture hormones to regulate weight and appetite. These hormones try to maintain the status quo – or the same state; this is also known as homeostasis.

Our bodies don't generally want to change. They like everything to stay the same. If we try to change things, our bodies will respond with compensation mechanisms, such as revving up our appetite hormones.

If we consistently consume less energy (in the form of food) than we expend through physical activity and basal metabolism (such as during a very low calorie diet), our bodies react by making us hungrier. This is why low calorie diets generally fail.

Leptin and ghrelin are the major hormones which regulate appetite. Leptin and ghrelin regulate the hunger center situated in a primitive part of your brain called the hypothalamus.

Ghrelin

The hormone ghrelin is secreted from the lining of the stomach. Your stomach will secrete a lot of ghrelin when you have not eaten for many hours to remind you that you need to eat NOW!

In summary, ghrelin increases hunger.

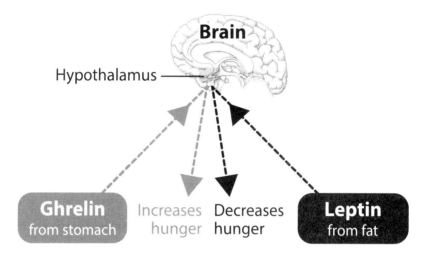

Ghrelin and leptin act on the brain via the hypothalamus.

Leptin

Leptin is made by our fat cells (adipose tissue) and is secreted into the circulatory system, where it travels to the hypothalamus. Leptin tells the hypothalamus that we have enough body fat, so we should eat less or stop eating.

Ideally the fatter you are the more leptin you make; thus you will eat less food and have a higher metabolic rate. Conversely, the less fat you have, the less leptin you make and your hunger will increase.

Thus leptin correlates to fat mass — the more fat you have, the more leptin you will produce.

Under normal conditions, leptin tells the brain that you are not hungry, and it tells the body to burn fat. Leptin decreases hunger and for weight loss — the more leptin the better!

However if leptin resistance develops, the whole control of hunger is disrupted - the result is a gnawing, constant hunger that cannot be satisfied.

Your leptin levels can be measured with a blood test when you are fasting (nothing but water for 12 hours).

- Ideal fasting leptin levels are between 4 to 6 ng/dL, but fasting leptin levels up to 9 ng/dL are considered normal.
- Leptin levels of over 10 ng/dL are considered to be too high.
- The majority of obese people have very elevated fasting levels of leptin from 20 to 40 ng/L.

Extremely low levels of fasting leptin are below 3, and are a sign of inadequate body fat; this can be due to malnutrition or intensive exercise.

The eating plan in this book will regulate your leptin levels to optimize weight loss. After 4 to 6 weeks on stage one of my diet, the vast majority of people have a large fall in their leptin levels, as well as their insulin levels. This is because they are no longer leptin or insulin resistant. The benefit is less hunger and fewer cravings.

How do the hunger signals get messed up?

Both Leptin and Ghrelin are designed to regulate hunger so that you stay in the healthy weight range – but the system is not perfect, as both these hormones and their signals get messed up with long term weight excess. As you become more and more overweight, and the longer you are overweight, the signals from these hunger hormones become more and more deranged and eventually stop working.

Leptin resistance

If the system worked perfectly you would think that fat people would somehow naturally stop eating or start losing weight once their leptin levels were high enough. Unfortunately, you can become leptin resistant; this is similar to the way that insulin resistance develops in overweight people.

If you are overweight, you can have a lot of fat making a lot of leptin, but the leptin doesn't work. The brain isn't listening to the leptin, so there is no drop in appetite and no increase in metabolism. Your brain might even think you're starving, because as far as it's concerned, there's not enough leptin. So you become even hungrier.

Leptin resistance is similar to insulin resistance

Insulin resistance occurs when there is excess insulin being produced (for example, with a diet high in sugar and refined carbohydrate), but the cells of your body and brain have stopped "listening" to insulin's effects.

Both insulin and leptin resistance seem to occur together in obese people but there are differences between the sexes. For example obese men who tend to have more internal belly fat (visceral fat) have higher insulin levels. Women who tend to have more fat under their skin have higher leptin levels.

There are a few possible explanations for how leptin resistance develops. One theory is that leptin cannot get to the hunger center in the hypothalamus because the proteins that transport it across the blood brain barrier are not working due to the build up of leptin in the cerebral spinal fluid that bathes the brain.

In summary once you are overweight, and the amount of fat you have reaches a critical amount, having slightly more body fat can mess up your appetite signals and actually make you hungrier.

Ghrelin

Leptin is a hormone that is a result of a build up of body fat; thus leptin is a long term regulator of body weight. Conversely ghrelin is the short term quick acting regulator of hunger - Hey I'm hungry now - when do we eat?

Your stomach makes ghrelin when it's empty. Ghrelin is secreted into the blood, crosses the blood-brain barrier, and goes to your hypothalamus, where it tells you that you are hungry. Ghrelin is high before you eat and low after you eat.

If you want to lose weight you want less ghrelin, so you don't get hungry. If you want to gain weight, say if you are very skinny, then you want more ghrelin — or at least you want it to stay high as you eat, so you'll want to eat more.

Both hormones regulate appetite and hunger, ideally to maintain homeostasis — in this case, keeping you adequately fed and in the healthy weight range. When you try to lose fat, your body will respond by making more ghrelin so that you get hungrier.

Bummer – as this presents a challenge for people trying to lose fat and keep it off and this can lead to the dreaded "yo-yo dieting" phenomenon.

The biggest hurdle dieters face is weight regain — and unless you have an eating plan to control your hunger hormones, dealing with rebound weight gain it is a daunting prospect.

The weight loss surgery known as Sleeve Gastrectomy works very well, as it removes the part of the stomach that produces ghrelin. Indeed after a Sleeve Gastrectomy many people never feel hungry again and massive amounts of weight loss are possible. But that could remove one of life's pleasures, but still for some morbidly obese people it could be lifesaving!

A study in the Journal of Clinical Endocrinology and Metabolism, 2010 Nov; 95(11):5037-44. Epub 2010, found interesting conclusions, which suggested that in obese people, leptin and ghrelin signals may not always work in ways that we expect. They concluded that obesity can disrupt normal appetite signaling.

The specialty of metabolic endocrinology is very complicated because no single hormone controls body composition, appetite and hunger. To be successful we need an eating plan that balances all our metabolic and hunger hormones and this book provides you with just that! Your individual hormonal profile may be relatively unique and needs to be considered.

There are proven things that you can do that will lead to a lasting change in body composition in a desirable way, namely less body fat and more muscle.

- Consume a diet that contains adequate protein and healthy natural fat so that your hunger hormones have a better chance of staying balanced and functional. The eating plan in this book is designed to do that and will keep your leptin, ghrelin and insulin levels under control
- Fine tune your thyroid hormones – see page 240
- Keep your liver healthy, as it helps to keep your hormones in balance
- Treat imbalances in sex hormones, especially progesterone deficiency and androgen excess
- Get adequate sleep, as a lack of sleep leads to more ghrelin and leptin resistance and thus weight gain
- Don't get discouraged, as it takes time to balance the hormones and the first 6 weeks are the most critical. Understand that when losing fat, you might be hungrier. That's normal and as long as you avoid carbohydrates and stick to safe foods you will cope
- Think positive and make a commitment to behavior change and regular exercise. Stay focused on your success. Stay focused on you. Ignore the negative thoughts that tell you that you will not succeed
- Stay in touch with my Weight Loss Detectives – they are highly trained and passionate about helping you. We've

helped thousands of people just like you lose weight and keep it off for good – see our videos of testimonials on www.liverdoctor.com

Fat makes hormones

Most people know that hormones are manufactured in our various glands, such as the pituitary gland, pancreas, the thyroid gland, the adrenal glands and the ovaries and testicles. However it may come as a surprise for you to learn that plenty of hormones are also manufactured in our fatty tissues.

Excessive amounts of upper level body fat produce more male hormones (androgens), which can increase insulin resistance and weight gain. Excessive production of androgens may cause "androgenization," resulting in excess facial and body hair, acne and thinning of the hair in a male pattern. This is what we find in many women with polycystic ovarian syndrome, especially if they carry a lot of weight in the upper body and abdomen.

Lower level body fat (below the waist) produces the female hormone called estrone, which if excessive, can increase fat deposits and cellulite in the hips, thighs and buttocks.

The hormone leptin is produced in our fat tissues. Long term obesity disrupts the action of leptin, so that we feel excessively hungry all the time.

Glucagon and Insulin

These two hormones are produced by the pancreas gland and together regulate sugar (glucose) and fat metabolism. These two hormones have a huge influence on your tendency to gain weight.

Glucagon has the opposite effect of insulin in the body. Glucagon stimulates the breakdown and burning of body fat. In contrast insulin promotes the storage of fat.

In summary the effects of the hormone glucagon are:

- It increases the burning of body fat stores for energy
- It converts fat and protein to glucose
- It pushes your metabolism into the fat burning zone
- It raises low blood glucose levels

Insulin exerts exactly the opposite effect to glucagon in the body, and thus it is better for those with a weight problem to find that their scale tips in the favor of glucagon and not insulin.

Thus glucagon and insulin are the two sides of the scale and need to be in balance for healthy metabolism.

What we eat has the most pronounced effect upon our insulin and glucagon ratio.

This is summarized in the chart below.

Food Category	Insulin Levels	Glucagon Levels
Carbohydrate	5	0
Protein	1	2
Fat	0	0
Protein and Fat	1	2
High protein and low carbohydrate	1	1
Carbohydrate and fat	4	0
High carbohydrate and low protein	9	1

From this chart you can see that dietary carbohydrate eaten by itself has a powerful effect in raising insulin levels. The adverse effect on insulin is at its worst when meals containing large amounts of refined carbohydrates with very low protein content are consumed.

My eating plan and supplement program has been designed to normalize body insulin levels, and maximize glucagon levels, so that these two crucial hormones of metabolism will remain in balance. Only then can fat burning take precedence over fat storage. Furthermore by correcting the balance of these two hormones we are treating the cause of Syndrome X. There will also be a correction in the other symptoms of Syndrome X – namely high blood pressure, high cholesterol levels and blood glucose instability. Another great benefit is that your cravings for carbohydrates will be much less, if not completely eradicated.

Adrenal Gland Dysfunction

The steroid hormone cortisol is made in the adrenal glands, and exerts a big effect on the metabolism of carbohydrates. Excessive levels of cortisol can cause a moon shaped face, fluid retention, raised blood sugar and weight gain around the abdomen. The levels of cortisol in the blood can be measured accurately with a simple blood test.

Prolonged mental stress can cause the adrenal glands to pump out excessive cortisol; this is one of the reasons that severe and prolonged stress can lead to weight gain. If stress is preventing you from losing weight, I recommend you undertake measures to get this under control as soon as possible. Worthwhile things to consider are a regular exercise program, getting to bed earlier, meditation, Yoga, Tai Chi, Pilates and clinical hypnotherapy. Taking a regular magnesium supplement can reduce stress.

Menopause and Weight Gain

Weight excess is common in women in during menopause and is commonly associated with Syndrome X and/or thyroid gland dysfunction. No matter what age you go through menopause, you will have fewer unpleasant symptoms if you have a regular exercise program, robust adrenal glands and a healthy liver. The liver breaks down (metabolizes) all the body's hormones, as well as any hormone replacement therapy that you may be taking. If the liver is sluggish or fatty, hormonal imbalances, hot flushes and sweats, insomnia and weight gain are far more common. The liver function can be improved with a liver formula such as Livatone and by increasing the amount of cooked and raw vegetables in the diet.

The adrenal glands are very important during and after menopause because they take over the role of the failed ovaries to a significant degree, and continue to produce significant amounts of testosterone and DHEA (dehydro-epiandrosterone). Women with healthy adrenal glands have much better energy levels, as well as a better sex drive. Supplements of magnesium, tyrosine, vitamin C and Adrenal Glandular Extract can boost adrenal function.

To avoid weight gain during menopause, choose hormone replacement therapy (HRT) that is bio-identical (more natural to your body), as this does not overwork the liver. Hormone creams containing mixtures of natural bio-identical hormones (such as estriol, estradiol, progesterone, DHEA and testosterone) or estrogen patches will bypass the liver. These types of hormones are absorbed into the blood stream through the skin and do not pass directly through the liver. For this reason they are far less likely to cause weight gain than hormone tablets.

In general by using lower doses of natural hormones that bypass the liver, we are able to avoid weight gain during menopause in women who are predisposed to obesity.

To keep your energy levels high so you can keep up the motivation to exercise, use super foods which are nutrient dense. These include brewer's yeast, spirulina, chia seeds, hemp seeds, freshly ground flaxseeds, walnuts, Brazil nuts, garlic, onions, radishes, and citrus fruits, freshly made raw vegetable juices, kelp, fresh sprouts, cold pressed oils, tahini or hummus, avocados and organic apple cider vinegar.

Hormonal case history

Rona came to see me complaining of abdominal weight gain, abdominal bloating, fatigue and facial hair. She was an apple shaped woman with all her weight excess in the trunk and abdomen, and had a large "liver roll" around her upper abdomen. Clinical assessment revealed that she had all the chemical imbalances of Syndrome X, with high triglycerides, low HDL cholesterol, and raised fasting insulin levels. An ultrasound scan of her upper abdomen revealed that she had a fatty liver. Her liver enzymes were slightly elevated, consistent with liver inflammation from fatty infiltration. She weighed 209 pounds (95 kilograms) and although she was quite tall, she looked very overweight. She had excess facial hair, which she controlled with regular waxing. Blood tests revealed high levels of male hormones with an elevated free testosterone level.

Rona had undergone a total hysterectomy with removal of both ovaries ten years previously. Thus not surprisingly, her levels of the female hormones estrogen and progesterone were non-existent. Rona needed natural estrogen and progesterone replacement therapy to balance her hormones, which would reduce her excessive male hormones. I prescribed these hormones in the form of a cream, which she rubbed into the inside skin of her upper arm twice daily. In her case I preferred the use of hormone creams instead of tablets or lozenges, as I did not want to over work her fatty liver. Rona was started on Glicemic Balance capsules to support insulin function and Livatone liver tonic, and instructed to follow a low carbohydrate gluten free eating plan.

Rona was accustomed to eating a lot of carbohydrates and her diet was deficient in vegetables, raw foods and protein. She did not find the change in her way of eating difficult, as once her insulin and leptin levels started to come down, she no longer felt so hungry

Six months after beginning her program Rona had lost 55 pounds (25 kilograms) with all the weight loss due to the reduction in excess fat from her trunk and abdomen. Her bloating had gone and she was able to wear belts and jeans again. Blood tests revealed normal levels of her male hormones, which was very desirable as this had reduced her facial hair. Her excessive levels *of male hormones had been coming from the fat in her upper body, and these male hormones had been increasing her insulin resistance and weight-gaining tendency.*

This case history shows how important it is to balance not only the insulin levels, but also any imbalances, which exist in other body hormones such as the sex hormones and thyroid hormones.

Premenstrual Syndrome and Weight Gain

The pre-menopausal ovaries have a cycle, which approximates 28 days, and is manifested by the development and release of a follicle (egg) from the ovary. Typically the egg is released from the ovary on day 14 of this cycle, and this is called ovulation. Immediately after ovulation the ovary starts to manufacture progesterone, which tones down your up-beat estrogen and makes the next 12 to 14 days pass at a slower pace. Progesterone will make you feel more relaxed and self-contented, so that this is a good time to meditate, think things through and pamper yourself.

The most testing zone of the monthly menstrual cycle is the 3 days before menstrual bleeding commences, because both estrogen and progesterone levels are dropping. This may cause unpleasant symptoms of the pre-menstrual syndrome, and is a time where your body and mind are more sensitive to all forms of stress. This tense zone is relieved by the onset of the menstrual bleeding, which causes a sense of physical and mental release once bleeding becomes established. During the premenstrual phase of the cycle, the drop in sex hormones may cause excess fluctuations in blood glucose levels. Some women get very strong cravings for carbohydrates and sugar during this phase and can easily put on several pounds of weight. To avoid premenstrual weight gain and fluid retention, you need to follow the eating plan in this book very closely during this phase of the cycle.

By eating regular first class protein, healthy fats and plenty of raw vegetables and fruits, you will find it much easier to prevent premenstrual weight gain. Taking a good liver tonic, magnesium and extra essential fatty acids can also help to prevent these problems.

Use natural progesterone cream to relieve premenstrual syndrome and to reduce weight gain around the hips and thighs. Synthetic hormones tend to cause weight gain.

If you need contraception, choose low dose feminine oral contraceptive pills such as Yaz or Zoely, which are less likely to cause weight gain than stronger contraceptive pills. If you have excess levels of male hormones (androgens), this can be controlled by taking medications that block the effect of these hormones. Suitable medications are Spironolactone or Cyproterone acetate, which prevent masculine effects of excessive male hormones such as facial hair and acne. In women with very high levels of male hormones, these medications can help with weight loss and appearance. Cyproterone acetate is more effective than Spironolactone.

Weight gain after childbirth

I have met many women who have complained of excess weight gain during and after pregnancy. Breast feeding your baby can help to keep your weight down; but in many women this is not enough to control their ballooning weight after childbirth.

The reasons for excessive weight gain during pregnancy and/or after childbirth include the following -

• The huge levels of hormones produced during pregnancy can increase the workload of the kidneys and liver, leading to fluid retention and an increased tendency to store fat. Women with a tendency to insulin resistance may find that they develop temporary diabetes of pregnancy, which is known as gestational diabetes. This worsening of insulin resistance often leads to a fat storing tendency.

• After the baby is born there is less personal time for exercise and sleep. Fatigue may result in less attention to meal preparation, making it easy to grab quick high carbohydrate snacks to keep energy levels up.

• Post natal depression may take away the motivation to follow a healthy eating plan and exercise program.

It is important to be aware of these risk factors and have a preventative plan to follow. Keep your liver and kidneys healthy by drinking plenty of water and raw vegetable juices. Have handy snacks available such as raw nuts, fresh raw coconut pieces, seeds, cheese and fruit, so you don't lose control and reach for the high sugar pick me ups. Keep the refrigerator stocked with plenty of high protein foods, such as cold roast beef and lamb, seafood (canned varieties of crab meat, sardines, salmon and tuna are excellent), and eggs. Boiled eggs are a complete food, providing all essential amino acids. Remember that protein depletion can lead to muscle loss and increased cravings for carbohydrates. Supplemental magnesium is very helpful for those with fluid retention and insulin resistance during pregnancy.

In many women with postnatal depression and weight gain, the use of natural progesterone cream or lozenges can help greatly. Natural progesterone is perfectly safe to take while breast-feeding and does not reduce the quantity of breast milk production.

It is important to act quickly if you find yourself gaining large amounts of weight after childbirth, as I have seen many women put on huge amounts of weight in a short period of time. It is then much harder to lose the weight, especially if you do nothing about it for several years.

Dr Cabot's Hormonal Advisory Service: This service provides information/referral for natural hormone therapy for post-natal depression, pre-menstrual syndrome and menopause.

Phone number: 623 334 3232 in the USA and 02 4655 8855 in Australia

Maggie's Case History

Maggie was typical of many women who come to see me trying to restore balance in their lives. For many women, physical and emotional balance can be elusive, especially since we cannot achieve one without the other. Maggie was 44 years old and had gained 46 pounds since she went through menopause 2 years ago. She was an apple shaped woman, carrying all her excessive weight in the abdominal area and had a roll of fat around her upper abdomen.

She forced herself to avoid eating, but even when she did this, she did not lose weight. Maggie just kept on gaining weight and had become extremely frustrated. Her doctor had given her high doses of the hormone estrogen in the form of Premarin tablets. These contain potent horse estrogens, as well as human estrogens. Maggie did not realize that she had a fatty liver, and her poor dysfunctional liver could not cope with the strong hormones she was taking. Understandably they had caused more weight gain, and Maggie was trapped in a vicious cycle of ever increasing weight.

After testing Maggie, I confirmed that she had a fatty liver, slightly high cholesterol and elevated fasting insulin, leptin and blood glucose levels. She felt hungry most of the time. Maggie was relieved to discover that she had a specific cause for her rapid weight gain - namely fatty liver and Syndrome X.

I stopped her Premarin tablets, and gave her a hormone cream containing natural human estrogen and progesterone. This would be much better for her overworked liver, which could now get on with its job of burning fat. Maggie loved protein and vegetables, so the Syndrome X eating plan was easy for her to follow. She found that avoiding high GI carbohydrates, such as crackers and breads, easily controlled her hunger. She had thought that these foods were helping her, but in Syndrome X, carbohydrates will increase the appetite.

Over a 6-month period Maggie lost 17.5 kg (39 pounds) and also considerably reduced her potbelly. She was able to fit into her old clothes and wear attractive belts again.

I find that many overweight women are taking inappropriate Hormone Replacement Therapy (HRT), which is aggravating their weight problem. It is not wise to take tablets containing strong or synthetic hormones, as these will increase the workload of the liver. I recommend hormone creams or patches containing natural estrogen and progesterone, as these are absorbed directly through the skin and bypass the liver. If we can reduce the workload of the liver it will be a more efficient fat burning organ.

John's Case History

John was undergoing treatment for male menopause (andropause) and was receiving injections of testosterone every 6 weeks. He was a busy man with his own business, and did not have much time to exercise or relax. He was apple shaped with abdominal obesity.

John had the chemical imbalance of Syndrome X with elevated triglycerides and fasting insulin levels. His high blood pressure was controlled with anti-hypertensive medication and he also took cholesterol-lowering drugs. At the age of 49 he found that the drug side effects were really destroying his sex life and slowing him down, so that his enjoyment of life was decreasing. He was frustrated especially as he had been told that the testosterone injections were going to make him feel wonderful. Indeed the injections had helped him initially, but his increasing weight was negating the short-lived benefits of the testosterone injections.

I started John on the Syndrome X eating plan, so that he had protein and vegetables at every meal and I increased his consumption of raw fruits and vegetables. He stopped drinking diet sodas and started drinking water. He was allowed 3 cups of black sugarfree coffee daily, as he really enjoyed his coffee. If he became hungry in between meals, he was allowed to nibble on nuts, cheese or a can of seafood. As a big man he had a huge appetite, so that healthy snacks were vital to see him through.

I also recommended LivaTone and Glicemic Balance to reduce his insulin resistance.

I stopped his testosterone injections and after 3 months I checked his blood levels of testosterone and DHEA. His levels were found to be at the lower limit of normal, so I prescribed a cream containing a combination of testosterone 60mg and DHEA 25mg daily.

Over a six month period, John lost 26 kg (59 pounds) and his waist to hip ratio reduced to 0.9. His blood pressure and cholesterol levels normalized, so that we were able to stop the medications he was taking. This was a great relief to John, as he hated the side effects and wanted to have a normal sex life again. He found that the hormone creams really helped him greatly, and did not produce the on-off effect that the injections had produced. He told me that he looked and felt 20 years younger, and his teenage son was delighted that his father was able to play sports with him once again. His wife was also very pleased to have her husband back, as she said, with "the old twinkle in his eyes!"

Assessing your weight

Simply by looking in the mirror it can be difficult to judge just how overweight or underweight you are. Perhaps you would prefer not to know!

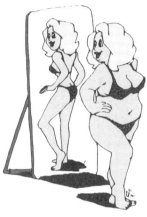

Never lose sight of your goal

A significant percentage of my patients do not allow me to weigh them on their first visit! Some people do not look as overweight as they really are. For example apple shaped people (Android body types) store a lot of fat within their body cavities and this fat is not visible. Conversely pear shaped people (Gynaeoid body types) carry their excess weight very visibly around their hips, buttocks and thighs. Lymphatic shaped people (Lymphatic body types) have a thicker layer of fat and fluid under their skin all over their body and they can look a lot more over weight than they really are.

Body Mass Index (BMI)

A useful graphic way of representing your weight can be done by plotting your weight on the next chart by drawing a line between your height on the left and your weight on the right. Your BMI is shown where the line intersects the scale in the middle.

Body weight can also be assessed by a ratio known as the Body Mass Index (BMI). For those not good at mathematics don't tune out, as it is really very simple! You can calculate your Body Mass Index by dividing your weight (in kilograms) by the square of your height (in meters).

$$\text{BMI} = \frac{\text{weight (kilograms)}}{\text{height x height (meters)}}$$

For example if you weigh 75 kilograms and are 1.69 meters (169 centimeters) tall, then your

$$\text{BMI} = \frac{75 \text{ kilograms}}{1.69 \text{ x } 1.69 \text{ meters}}$$

$$= \frac{75}{2.856}$$

$$\text{Your BMI} = 26.26$$

To convert pounds to kilograms, divide the pounds by 2.2
- for example 154 pounds divided by 2.2 = 70 kilograms

To convert inches to meters, multiply the inches by 0.0254
- for example 68 inches multiplied by 0.0254 = 1.727 meters.

If you don't like equations, you can easily work out your BMI from the scales on our chart. *See over.*

To use the scale, place a ruler between your weight (undressed) and your height (without shoes). Then read your BMI on the middle scale.

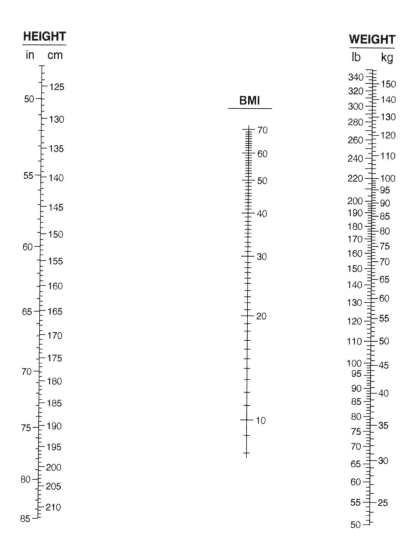

BMI Scale

BMI Table	
BMI less than 18	lean to underweight
BMI 19 to 25	desirable for women
BMI 20 to 26	desirable for men
BMI 26 to 30	overweight
BMI 31 to 40	obesity
BMI over 40	severe obesity

Weight can vary by 2 to 4 pounds over one day, due to fluid retention, constipation, a full bladder, sweating and hormonal changes. Weighing yourself once a week is sufficient, less frustrating and less prone to small errors. When weighing yourself choose the same time of the day, wearing no clothes.

What should the body fat percentage of your total body weight be?

Age	Percentage of Body Fat
Women	
Up to 30 years	20 to 26%
31 to 40 years	21 to 27%
41 to 50 years	22 to 28%
Over 50 years	22 to 31%

Age	Percentage of Body Fat
Men	
Up to 30 years	12 to 18%
31 to 40 years	13 to 19%
Over 40 years	13 to 21%
Over 50 years	22 to 31%

Note: Women whose body fat percentage falls below 15% may have problems with their body's production of sex hormones. This can cause infertility and lead to absent menstruation and osteoporosis.

Obstacles to Successful Weight Loss

Weight Loss Plateaus

The "weight loss plateau" can affect anyone who is making their best efforts while on a weight loss diet. It is generally misunderstood but is not to be feared. The "weight loss plateau" can be described as a flattening out in the weight loss curve while following a weight loss diet. During this flattening of the curve, weight loss ceases for a variable period of time but generally for 2 to 4 weeks.

A weight loss plateau is the dangerous time when many people become frustrated and falsely believe that the eating plan they are following is not working. You are wrong it is working!

During a weight loss plateau the scales are your worst enemy – beware, as the scales have set many dieters up for failure!

During this plateau phase, the desired changes in your metabolism and appetite control hormones are taking place, even though you cannot see them and you may stop losing weight.

Be patient as it takes time to -

- Reduce insulin and leptin levels
- Remove unhealthy fat from the liver

All this will be happening while you are following my eating plan and using appropriate supplements, but you may not see these things occurring behind the scenes. While your body is busy achieving this metabolic correction, there may be times when weight loss stops, but this is only temporary. Indeed weight loss plateaus may be necessary lulls in your rate of weight loss. If you become impatient and revert to eating excess carbohydrates during a plateau phase, you will undo weeks of beneficial changes, not to mention your own hard work. Indeed by jumping off the eating plan while in a plateau phase, you may become a yo-yo dieter. If you do go on a binge of wrong foods, don't despair – just exercise it off, but don't wait more than a few days.

So my message is just hang in there! Relax - the desired changes are happening inside your liver, your fat cells, and your appetite hormones - within a few weeks weight loss will resume at a normal healthy pace.

If you do fall off the wagon, do not freak out and lose your inspiration. Just get back onto the eating plan, but remember it may take a few weeks before you see the weight coming off. However your energy levels should improve within a few days of recommencing the eating plan in this book.

Some people have been overweight for many years; they may find it extremely difficult to commence losing weight, or they may stay in a weight loss plateau for too long. If this is you and you are becoming impatient there are several things that you can try -

- For four weeks have meals comprised ONLY of the following - red or white meat, poultry, seafood, cheese, plain unflavored yoghurt and eggs combined with salad vegetables and/or cooked green leafy vegetables. Avoid all starchy vegetables such as potato, carrots, swede, turnip and pumpkin. This diet is virtually free of carbohydrate and will put you into a state of fat burning or ketosis. See page 303. Your insulin levels will plummet and after several days you will not feel hungry. Those who are pregnant, or those with diabetes type 1 or kidney disease are not able to follow this strict regime. Type 2 diabetics can follow it under supervision from a registered health care practitioner.
- Go on a vegetable juice fast for 7 days. Your body will go into a state of fat burning and you will probably have ketones in your urine by day 2 of the juice fast. The presence of ketones in the urine indicates that

you are breaking down your body fat and using it for energy. This state of ketosis is only temporary and is not a problem as long as you are not pregnant or diabetic. Check with your own health care professional if you are not sure you can try a juice fast.

- Go on a liquid diet for 7 days, consisting of a sugar free protein powder drink (such as Synd-X Slimming Protein Powder) mixed in sugar free milk (dairy, coconut, almond or soy), raw vegetable juices and vegetable soups or broths. You may have any of these liquids whenever you feel hungry.
- Take supplements to reduce insulin and leptin resistance – these consist of magnesium and Glicemic Balance capsules.

Depression and Stress

Depression and other emotional imbalances can lead to problems with body weight, from weight loss to weight gain. This is because the chemical imbalance existing within the brain of depressed people, may affect the appetite control center in the brain. Some people need to overeat to fill up a perceived emptiness inside, and food becomes their solace. Others will turn to food if they are anxious, stressed and over pressured. Some of these people may become obsessive-compulsive eaters.

If you feel that depression and/or stress may be sabotaging your weight loss efforts you can look into several options -

- Support groups such as Over-Eaters Anonymous or Weight Watchers can be very helpful.
- Join a club with physical activities such as a tennis club, bushwalking club or a swimming club. Aqua-aerobics, swimming or just walking in a swimming pool can be the best exercise for overweight persons, as it does not stress the joints.
- Have a regular therapeutic massage to relieve pent up physical and emotional stresses.

- Go for a walk each morning with a group of friends or your dog.
- Seek counseling from a psychotherapist or psychologist to work on the reasons why you crave comfort foods in excess amounts.
- Consult a clinical hypnotherapist to learn to control your subconscious reasons for overeating; this is often very successful.
- Use meditation and positive affirmations.

If the depression is severe enough for your doctor to classify it as a "clinical depression" you may need to take anti-depressant medication. Anti-depressant drugs will not put on weight if you stay away from excess carbohydrates and keep exercising. For more help see my books *Help for Depression and Anxiety* and *Want to lose weight but hooked on Food?*

Low Blood Sugar Levels (Hypoglycemia)

Low blood glucose (Hypoglycemia) is a common cause of strong cravings for sugar and carbohydrates. Thus it is important to prevent hypoglycemia. The best way to do this is to ensure that you are eating first class protein at least 3 times daily. If you are busy, you can use a sugar free protein powder drink, such as Synd-X Slimming Protein Powder or protein snacks such as canned seafood, cheese and olives or nuts and seeds. Tasty nuts are macadamias, pecans, cashews, walnuts and Brazil nuts; these are convenient and have a significant amount of healthy fats to satisfy you. For this reason they tend to suppress the appetite. These protein foods are very low in carbohydrate and will help to prevent erratic fluctuations in blood glucose levels.

Avocados are also excellent to eat if you have blood sugar problems. Avocados are high in healthy mono-unsaturated fats, and low in carbohydrate. Foods high in mono-unsaturated fats have been shown to reduce insulin and leptin resistance. Avocados are healthy and filling, and are delicious if you fill their cavity with seafood or white cheese and olives. They also taste very nice with sun-dried tomatoes.

If you must have something sweet, try eating fresh fruit with dark chocolate or make a shake with the Synd-X Slimming protein Powder, coconut milk and berries.

Food addiction

The taste of foods high in sugar or gluten can be addictive, especially if you have severe drops in your blood glucose levels. Once you become accustomed to eating high sugar foods on a regular basis, your body will come to expect them regularly, so it is best to stop as soon as possible.

Sometimes the cravings for sweets or gluten can become overbearing and you need to have some strategies to overcome these cravings.

To reduce cravings I recommend -

- **A good quality protein powder.** I recommend a powder designed for Syndrome X called Synd-X Slimming Protein Powder; use this when you get a craving for something sweet. The full range of amino acids in Synd-X Powder will help to stabilize blood glucose levels and increase energy. The addition of extra L - glutamine in this powder can act as an alternative fuel for the brain, which means the brain does not rely so much on blood glucose for energy. Synd-X Protein Powder also contains supplemental taurine and chromium picolinate, which helps to stabilize blood glucose levels. Simply mix the protein powder in unsweetened milk, and make a shake in the blender. Coconut milk contains short chain fats known as MCTs which are easily metabolized by the brain for energy and is an aid to weight loss.

- **Salty foods** - the craving for sugar and refined carbohydrates can often be replaced with salty foods. Salt does not cause fat gain. Suitable examples are salted peanuts or other salted nuts, anchovies, sun dried tomatoes, olives, capers and salty cheeses.

- **The amino acid tyrosine**. Tyrosine is required for the manufacture of important brain neurotransmitters; these include dopamine and noradrenalin, which impact greatly on mood and appetite.

  Low dopamine or noradrenalin levels have been linked with –

  - Food cravings (particularly for carbohydrate)
  - Excessive appetite
  - Reduced ability to experience pleasure and satisfaction
  - Reduced concentration and mental drive

A study carried out by Dr Alan Gelenberg of the Harvard Medical School showed clearly that a lack of the amino acid tyrosine resulted in a deficiency of the brain transmitter noradrenalin. This deficiency occurred at certain locations in the brain, which relate specifically to mood disorders. Tyrosine can be an excellent and safe natural antidepressant and in general exerts a stimulating effect. Tyrosine can lift the mood and improve concentration and mental drive. Sometimes tyrosine is referred to as a "mood food" because it is a protein supplement that can improve mood.

Tyrosine supplementation may provide the following benefits:

- Improved concentration and alertness
- More motivation
- Increased ability to experience satisfaction and pleasure
- Reduction in depression
- Reduced appetite in those with eating disorders

Some people battling with drug, food and/or alcohol addiction find that tyrosine helps them to detoxify and reduce their cravings. It has been used successfully to help people overcome a cocaine addiction.

How to take tyrosine

Tyrosine is best taken away from food, two or three times daily. The recommended dose is 1 to 2 grams, two or three times daily. Some people may need higher doses than this so work with your health care practitioner to increase the dose if lower doses are ineffective.

Contraindications to taking tyrosine - Tyrosine supplements must not be used by people taking monoamine oxidase inhibitor (MAOI) medications. Tyrosine can be safely used by people taking the modern day and commonly prescribed SSRI anti-depressants.

If you have a malignant melanoma don't take tyrosine unless you check with your doctor first.

For more information contact the Health Advisory Service on 623 334 3232 in the USA or 02 4655 8855 in Australia.

Pathways of neurotransmitter production in the brain

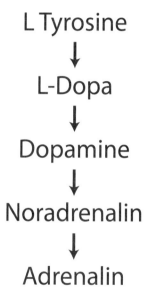

L Tyrosine
↓
L-Dopa
↓
Dopamine
↓
Noradrenalin
↓
Adrenalin

Chocolate is special

Some people need chocolate more than love and cannot exist without any chocolate in their lives. In all honesty I cannot think of a substitute for the experience of chocolate. I recently met a woman who suffered with obesity and

Syndrome X, and consumed seven family sized blocks of chocolate a week!

If you are a chocolate addict and must have chocolate, I suggest that you treat yourself to chocolate once a week, but do not eat the family size block and stick to a smaller chocolate bar or dark chocolate. There are good brands of chocolate available that are sweetened with stevia or sugar alcohols and are low in carbohydrate.

Lack of Exercise

Previous generations walked an average of 15,000 steps per day. The average office worker now walks only 3,000 steps daily. It is important to understand that exercise does not just burn calories; it will fundamentally change your metabolism so that you are able to turn fat into muscle.

We all know that regular exercise will assist in increasing the metabolic rate and weight loss. However some people don't enjoy exercise and prefer to watch someone else exercise! Furthermore if you are overweight, you may feel uncomfortable about wearing a swim suit or exercise shorts, or mixing with slim people at the local gym. One thing that I have found easy to do is to put on some music at home and dance around the lounge room. You can also exercise with a small pair of hand weights while you dance, or follow along with an exercise video, in the privacy of your own home. The hand weights will tone and firm the arms, which may become flabby with weight loss. Some people find it useful to acquire the help of a personal trainer, although this can be expensive, but is generally well worth the expense. Your exercise routine should be done regularly to gradually improve your fitness level. Pedometers, available in electronics stores, are a good way to try to get your 10,000 steps per day.

If you fall into the very over-weight range, the best exercise to start with is gentle swimming, an exercise bike or Tai Chi or Pilates. Walking or jogging may damage your joints, especially the knees and hips, or aggravate back pain if you are very overweight. As you lose weight, more strenuous exercises can be started and this is where a personal trainer can make a huge difference.

Be on the look-out for opportunities to exercise, such as getting off the bus a few stops earlier, taking the stairs instead of the elevator, leaving your car at home, or stopping for a walk in the park at lunch breaks. Some days you may feel like putting it off, but try to force yourself to overcome laziness because the results are many times worth the effort. The more you exercise the better you will look and feel. If you burn up 250 calories (1050 kJ) daily with exercise, this would result in a weekly weight loss of ½ pound. If you burn up 500 calories (2100 kJ) daily with exercise, this would result in a weekly weight loss of just over one pound.

Activity	Calories Burned Per Min.
Very Light e.g. dusting or slow walking	2 (8.4kJ)
Moderate e.g. brisk walking, energetic gardening or scrubbing the floor	3.5-7 (14.7-29.4kJ)
Heavy e.g. running, aerobics swimming laps, rowing or weight training	>7.5 (>31.5kJ)

See our exercise video on https://www.sandracabot.com/exercises-to-keep-you-fit-part-1/ to see the techniques of naturopath and personal trainer Vicky Jane Spencer where she demonstrates exercises with Marcelle Mogg who has lost nearly 50 kilograms (110 lbs) in weight on our program.

The fitter you are the lower your resting heart rate is, which means that you can deal better with stress, without such a large build-up of chemical by-products in your system. The best exercise is a constant rhythmical type, where you are using the large muscle groups at an intensity that increases your heart rate to 60 per cent of your maximum heart rate.

This is called your target heart rate. It is necessary to achieve your target heart rate, if you want to increase your metabolic rate, and so increase the rate at which you burn up excess fat.

To find your maximum heart rate –

• Subtract your age from 220

To find your target heart rate -

• Multiply the above figure (220 minus your age) by 0.6

For example, if you are 40 years old, your maximum heart rate = 220 minus 40 = 180 beats per minute. Your target heart rate = 180 x 0.6 = 108 beats per minute. By reaching your target heart rate during exercise, you will increase your metabolic rate.

To reduce cellulite you should leave no longer than 48 hours between each session of exercise. You can work out for anything between thirty to sixty minutes a session, three to five times a week. Ideally, you could do five, thirty-minute sessions per week, as that would keep your metabolic rate up and running, therefore preventing the build up of cellulite.

Massage and hydrotherapy are also excellent in helping to stimulate lymphatic drainage and reduce cellulite.

During exercise, skeletal muscle needs energy, and gets it by metabolizing glucose and muscle glycogen. This is a very effective way to burn calories. In sedentary people, skeletal muscle cells demonstrate insulin resistance, and exercise can help to reduce insulin resistance. Exercise will regulate your desire for food and speed up your weight loss.

Colin's Case history

Colin was a typical example of a man who was addicted to carbohydrates. He started his day with black coffee laden with 3 teaspoons of sugar, and tried to avoid eating, as he thought this would help him to lose weight. He then went to his office job and found that by 11am he started to crave something sweet. He went to the snack machine where he obtained a packet of chips, a coke and a chocolate bar. He said the sugar tasted great going down, but once it hit his stomach he felt nauseated.

Lunchtime consisted of a large plate of pasta covered with a creamy sauce and washed down by another coke. The pasta gave him a big dose of carbohydrate and filled him up until around 3pm. By this time he needed more coffee laden with sugar and a sweet biscuit. On his way home from work he thought of sugar and knew every snack bar on the way home from work. He could not resist the temptation to buy some sugary donuts and more soft drink. By 7pm he felt exhausted, and usually made himself a quick meal of toast and jam or toast and cheese. His diet was very poor, being deficient in protein, vegetables and essential fatty acids.

Colin felt quite hopeless about losing weight and had tried everything from gastric banding to laxatives and many low-fat low-calorie diets. He believed it was his fault and that he would never be able to lose his addiction to carbohydrates.

When Colin came to see me he was 130 kilograms (286 pounds) and was 5 foot 10 inches (1.75 meters) tall. He had a lot of weight accumulated around his trunk and abdominal area, and a roll of fat around the upper abdomen which indicated a fatty liver. His legs were reasonably slim and muscular, and his hips were narrow. He really had upper level body obesity, and was the Android Body Type.

Blood tests revealed that Colin had Syndrome X, as his fasting triglycerides, LDL cholesterol and insulin levels were all elevated. A 2-hour Glucose Tolerance Test (GTT) showed that he had temporarily elevated levels of blood glucose, which then became abnormally low after 3 hours. At this time he had a marked craving for sugar and felt weak and shaky.

I explained to Colin that he had a chemical imbalance known as Syndrome X, which was 90% of the reason that he was addicted to carbohydrates and sugar. He was relieved to know that there *was a medical problem that made him crave the wrong foods, and also kept him too exhausted to exercise.*

I started Colin on my eating plan so that he was having regular protein and adequate fat. He began having things like eggs and bacon or an omelette for breakfast, a large salad and chicken for lunch, and seafood or meat with vegetables and salad for his evening meal. While he was at work he kept a supply of raw nuts and seeds, cheese, olives and his Synd- X Slimming Protein powder handy. He would use these things to snack on when the sugar cravings hit him.

This gave Colin more confidence, as he now had a very specific way of eating to put himself back in control of his blood sugar and hunger hormones. After the first week he phoned me, saying that he had not lost any weight but felt more energetic and had not had one craving for sugar. Indeed he was wondering if he was eating too much, as the salads and vegetables took much longer to eat than his previous foods, and really seemed to fill him up. After the second week he started to lose weight steadily from his abdomen, and lost the bloated feeling he had always had around his abdomen. One thing he found very handy to stave off carbohydrate cravings was canned crab meat and avocado. He took these things to work, and had them in the mid-afternoon, if his blood sugar dropped; this kept him craving-free until his evening meal. He loved the taste of crab meat and thought it was a real treat being able to eat shellfish as he desired. For years he had thought that he must avoid shellfish, as it would raise his cholesterol levels. Little did he know that the healthy fats found in raw coconut flesh, shellfish and avocado, were a great weapon against his obesity and insulin resistance. It was sugar and refined carbohydrates that were causing his metabolic problem, and not protein or fat.

In total Colin lost 38 kilograms (84 pounds) over 18 months, and it all came off from his abdomen and trunk area. An ultrasound scan of his liver showed that it was no longer fatty and his blood tests were now all normal. He no longer had Syndrome X. Now that his body chemistry was back to normal, he no longer craved refined carbohydrates and sugar, which to him was utterly amazing. When he became hungry he thought of protein, healthy natural fats and vegetables. He also enjoyed the flavor of the "Synd-X Protein Powder", which he used regularly to keep his energy levels high.

Poor preparation results in poor performance

The 5 P's = Prior Preparation Prevents Poor Performance. . . . and be POSITIVE!!!

Here is a testimonial from a patient who tried the HCG Diet

My experience goes like this . . .

Being fat sux. I am the queen of excuses as to why I cannot diet and/or lose weight. I have tried most diets and they never work – often because of self sabotage on my part.

I flew from Central Queensland to Sydney to see Weight Loss Detective Kylie McCarthy. I decided before I booked the flight that this diet was going to work and work for me.

Instead of making excuses I put into practice the 5 P's. Prior to starting the diet, I got organized.

A few things that helped me out were -

- Digital scales to weigh protein. I bought chicken breast, steak, fish etc once a week and weighed and bagged up protein in 100gram (3.5oz) lots and put them in the freezer. In the morning I would take out what I needed for that day I would also cook and freeze chicken breasts in 100gram bags to have for lunch each day when I was at work
- Digital scales to weigh myself
- Tape measure
- George Foreman grill

- When I went out for 'drinks' I would be the designated driver and stick to soda water
- Have non-food related events planned. I would get my nails painted for example
- Buy new skin care products that are oil free
- Plan events - I went away for a weekend camping and took the George Forman grill and vegetables
- Being in a shopping center and being caught short – I would go to the Supermarket and buy a punnet of strawberries or an apple
- Read inspiring or funny books
- Organise the pantry and fridge
- Only tell people that will be supportive
- Get mentally prepared. The HCG Diet is ONLY 3 to 6 weeks
- Set up appointments with your weight loss detective
- Write down any questions you may have

By being prepared I had given myself the best chance to succeed. There were some days that were tougher than others of course, but this really helped. I stuck to the HCG diet and drops for 6 weeks. Although I didn't lose as much weight as I had hoped, I still feel 100% better than I did before the HCG diet, and, I am going to do it again. I sleep better, I don't snore, I don't have heartburn, I've dropped a dress size, I feel stronger within myself and I am more confident. Rome was not built in a day and with the right help we never have to give up. For information about HCG diets go to www.drsandracabotclinics.com.au/hcg-diet/

Frequently asked questions

Do very high protein diets work?

Many of these diets don't work because they do not give enough emphasis on improving the liver function, which means that in the long term, they will not be as effective in weight control and achieving optimal health.

High protein high fat diets (with very low carbohydrate intake) will help with initial weight loss because they reduce glucose and insulin levels and often put you into a state of ketosis (fat burning). However if they do not contain enough vegetables you can run into metabolic problems.

This is because of the following:

- The liver and kidneys may become overworked by having to process and eliminate large amounts of protein. Dietary protein is broken down into ammonia, which is processed by the liver and turned into urea and creatinine, which are waste products of metabolism. Urea and creatinine must be eliminated by the kidneys via the urine. Have you ever noticed that your urine gets a strong ammonia type of smell the day after consuming a meal with very high amounts of animal protein? This is because of the high content of ammonia, urea and creatinine waste products in the urine from eating so much protein in one hit.

Weight loss is not just about rapid loss; it is about taking off the weight and keeping it off. Furthermore we are trying to improve our general health and longevity and to achieve this, healthy liver and kidney function is vital. This is why balance is so important, and in my eating program you will achieve the correct balance of nutrients to stimulate fat burning.

Many high protein diets allow you to eat lots of preserved and processed fatty meats and deep fried meats, which contain damaged fats. This is not a healthy way of eating for life extension.

In my eating plan I allow you to eat a reasonable amount of saturated fat from specific foods, as long as it is fresh, not deep-fried and not processed. Remember that your brain contains a lot of saturated fat – 25% of the weight of your brain comes from pure cholesterol.

Why don't very low-fat low-calorie diets work?

These diets do not work because they are too low in the good fats, and too high in carbohydrates.

I have seen many people become yo-yo dieters on low-calorie diets because they are consuming too much sugar or artificial sweeteners found in such diet foods – an example is a sweet low fat yoghurt.

Temporary weight loss may occur because the daily calories are low, but the very low caloric intake causes the metabolic rate to slow down, so that when you come off the diet, your metabolic rate is at an all time low. So once you begin to eat normally and increase the calories, you will gain weight more rapidly than ever before.

Dietary protein and fat does not require much insulin to process, whereas carbohydrates do. A diet predominantly obtained from low fat high GI carbohydrates will increase insulin levels, and remember it is the insulin excess that makes you fat!

Low-fat low-calorie diets usually cause instability of blood glucose levels, which results in fatigue and cravings for more carbohydrates. It is the fatigue and cravings that will sabotage your efforts to stay with a healthy way of eating.

I had one patient who had been trying to lose weight for 25 years on low calorie diets and was a typical yo-yo dieter. She could not stay on a diet for longer than 2 weeks because of extreme tiredness and cravings, which made her become obsessed with sweet foods. She would hide these foods so she could not get at them and avoided socializing. She had come to accept chronic fatigue as a way of life, and gave up the idea of ever being slim and healthy.

I started her on my eating program and she lost her cravings and had more energy than she had experienced in years. She started to lose weight around her abdomen and lost her bloated feeling, which gave her a renewed sense of hope. A few weeks later as her confidence returned, she attended a weekend conference, and decided to enjoy the lunch of high carbohydrate foods provided. She thought that surely only one episode of eating high carbohydrate - refined foods would not cause her any problems. In the middle of the afternoon her blood glucose dropped during a lecture presentation, and she was woken up by the lady sitting next to her, as her loud snoring was making it difficult for others to hear the lecture. She was mortified and realized that her metabolism was profoundly affected by what she ate. If she had been able to eat protein foods such as fresh meats, eggs, nuts, beans and seeds along with vegetables and salad, she would have been able to enjoy the seminar and avoid acute embarrassment.

Why is Synd-X Protein powder different to other weight loss protein powders?

Synd-X Slimming Protein powder is extremely low in carbohydrates and extremely high in protein.

It provides a source of complete protein in a convenient and easily digested form. It is great for a quick energy burst, and to sustain you during hunger pangs in between meals. If you are busy, or just feeling lazy, you can make a complete meal out of "Synd-X Protein Powder" and some fruit.

I have found that whey protein concentrate is the most effective protein supplement for those with a weight problem.

Soy or pea protein is not such a high quality protein as whey protein concentrate is. Those who are highly allergic to dairy products and/or lactose intolerant may not be able to use whey protein.

I prefer protein powders that are unsweetened, or sweetened with the natural herb Stevia, rather than artificially sweetened powders.

Synd-X Slimming Protein Powder contains the following -

- Whey protein concentrate is its main ingredient and this supplies all amino acids
- Taurine, which is essential for healthy liver function and fat metabolism
- Glutamine, which acts as a fuel for the brain and reduces cravings for sweets and alcohol. It is also useful for digestive disorders and is able to increase lean muscle mass and decrease the body fat percentage, probably by its beneficial effect upon blood glucose control
- Chromium picolinate, which helps to reduce insulin resistance and stabilize blood glucose levels
- Stevia a naturally sweet herb with zero calories and zero carbohydrate content

Synd-X Protein powder can be used in the following ways -

- To make a pleasant drink by itself in between meals, or as a quick breakfast – add some LSA, chia seeds or hemp seeds and berries and plain yogurt for great taste.
- To make a "smoothie" with added fruit (such as banana, passion fruit, strawberries, mango or blackberries etc.) and ground flaxseed in a blender.
- To make a tropical "smoothie" on a hot summer day - try adding some coconut milk or coconut cream, small amounts of fresh fruits (such as kiwi fruit, mango, passion fruit, papaya or banana), a few drops of vanilla essence - blend all together in blender and serve on the rocks - delicious!
- To sprinkle over cereals or desserts to increase their protein content

Does weight loss surgery work?

In my experience weight loss surgery has different results in different people and is not a panacea for weight loss.

Weight loss surgery is known as bariatric surgery and consists of –

- Gastric banding
- Sleeve gastrectomy
- Gastric bypass

I have seen many patients who have had gastric banding who have had only limited success. This is because they continued to eat a high carbohydrate diet. It is easy to eat a diet high in soft drinks, alcohol, ice cream and chocolate after stomach surgery. These patients did not follow a healthy lifestyle and still kept their negative self beliefs. The majority of these patients regained around 80% of the weight they initially lost – very disappointing. Some of them experienced complications such as abdominal pain and vomiting due to the band eroding the stomach or becoming displaced and required surgery to remove the band and scar tissue.

The sleeve gastrectomy is generally more successful than gastric banding, as it not only reduces the amount of food that can be eaten, it also removes part of the stomach that produces the hunger hormone called ghrelin. Thus after this surgery patients do not feel hungry and resist temptation well. They usually lose massive amounts of weight initially and reverse their diabetes. For the very obese this surgery can be life saving. I have been impressed by some of the results obtained by sleeve gastrectomy. I have also seen patients who regained much of their lost weight after sleeve gastrectomy for the same reasons that gastric banding can fail. In some cases the patients resorted to a liquid diet high in sugar and other carbohydrates and thus they developed Syndrome X again. Thus the surgery did not fix their metabolic problem. After sleeve gastrectomy the small sleeve of remaining stomach can gradually expand so that the stomach becomes much larger meaning that they can resume eating larger meals.

So in summary I would only recommend bariatric surgery as part of a holistic program which incorporates low carbohydrate eating, exercise and continued psychological support and counseling.

Should I avoid eggs and coconut?

Eggs are high in cholesterol and if we listen to some nutritionists and the popular press we often find that eggs are portrayed as unhealthy, especially for those with high blood cholesterol levels or heart problems. I do not agree with this opinion because eggs contain high concentrations of many valuable nutrients and are a great food to eat for losing weight. Moreover most of the studies that showed eggs raised cholesterol were done using powdered eggs. Powdered eggs contain oxidized or damaged cholesterol (known as oxy-cholesterol), and this has a different effect in the body than pure fresh cholesterol. Other studies have found that hard-boiled eggs do not raise cholesterol levels in the majority of patients. A study done at the University of California found that the consumption of two boiled eggs daily did not increase cholesterol levels at all. The reason why eggs are health promoting, is that eggs have a high content of lecithin. Lecithin has been proven to lower cholesterol and helps to keep it soluble, so that it does not form plaques in the blood vessels. Eggs are also high in the sulphur bearing amino acids taurine, cysteine and methionine, which are required by the liver to regulate bile production and detoxification.

Eat as many eggs as you like as they will help you to lose weight and reduce cravings. If you eat more cholesterol your liver will make less cholesterol and this is a self regulating process.

You can consume a sensible and satisfying amount of cholesterol-containing foods such as cheese, butter, cream and eggs; make sure that they are fresh, so that their contained fats are not oxidized.

Remember that the liver makes 80% of the body's cholesterol, and cholesterol levels are regulated automatically by a HEALTHY liver. If you consume a little more cholesterol on one day, the liver will not manufacture as much of its own cholesterol, and things will balance out nicely. Liver function has a much greater effect upon cholesterol levels, than does a modest consumption of healthy foods containing cholesterol.

Coconut is another much maligned food and indeed is unworthy of its jaded reputation. I personally prefer Asian sauces, especially delicious Thai recipes, which are made with coconut milk or coconut cream, to creamy sauces made with dairy products. I find that coconut milk and/or cream sauces are light, and do not produce mucus in the body. I have never found that fresh coconut flesh, coconut milk or coconut sauces have caused high cholesterol levels or weight problems in my patients. Coconuts and their milk do not contain any cholesterol.

Can I eat dairy products on this program?

In general dairy products are suitable during a weight loss program as they are high in protein and contain healthy saturated fats and are low in carbohydrate. This is provided they do not contain added sugar. Everyone is different, which means that some people will have individual intolerances to foods and this means that some trial and error will be involved. Most people are able to consume dairy products with no problems. Others will have problems from eating dairy products, such as recurrent infections of the sinuses, excess mucus or irritable bowel syndrome if they are lactose intolerant. Some people with autoimmune disease are unable to tolerate dairy products and it is worth going on a dairy free diet for 4 months to see the difference.

Dairy products consist of animal milks and their derivatives, namely butter, cheese, cream and yoghurt. Most commercially available ice-cream and dairy chocolates are usually high in sugar. You can make your own ice cream containing dairy cream, coconut cream, raw eggs, Nature Sweet Sugar Substitute or stevia and fresh fruit. You need a blender or ice cream maker.

How can I help my child to lose weight?

Not infrequently I receive pleas for help from mothers whose young children have a fatty liver. Thirty years ago it was extremely rare to find fatty livers in children, as this condition was usually seen in older persons who had a long history of alcohol abuse or obesity.

Indeed not long ago I received a phone call from one of my naturopaths, regarding a mother who was highly distressed about her 9year-old son who had a severe case of fatty liver. It was so severe that she had been told her son would require a liver transplant. It is incredible to think that such a young boy would be suffering with a fatty liver. When I spoke to this woman I asked her about the child's diet. She told me that her son hated eating anything raw, and would not eat any fruits or vegetables at all. His diet mainly consisted of bread and margarine, chips, sweet cereals, hamburgers and snack foods high in sugar and hydrogenated vegetable oils. He would eat a little meat, but preferred fatty hamburger meat and mincemeat, and would not drink water. He only drank soft fizzy drinks, so she had started to give him diet drinks full of aspartame. The boy was very overweight and carried most of the weight in the abdominal area. It is hard for children like this who have been brought up on sugar and artificial fats, as their taste buds have become distorted.

Another case history of interest involves a mother in the USA, who E-mailed me for help with her six year old daughter who was 48 inches (1.2 meters) tall and weighed 85 pounds (40 kilograms). This child carried her excess weight in the trunk and abdomen, and was found to have elevated liver enzymes. She was tested for all sorts of liver disease and was eventually found to have a fatty liver on an ultrasound scan. This very young child was found to have the chemical imbalances of Syndrome X – namely elevated triglycerides and insulin levels, although thankfully her blood glucose levels were still within normal limits. She did suffer with the adult problem of heartburn due to reflux of stomach acids caused by her enlarged fatty liver pressing upon her stomach. According to her mother, her daughter's favorite foods were ice cream, salty chips and crackers. The child's diet was analyzed by a dietitian, and was found to be too high in carbohydrates (75% of her daily calories) and too low in protein.

This mother started her daughter on the eating plan in my book *Fatty Liver – You can reverse it*, as her specialist approved this diet as very helpful for her child's condition.

Children should not be placed on a calorie-restricted diet unless supervised by a dietitian or doctor.

Helpful things that you can do to help your child include:

- Provide your child with a structured meal and snack plan
- Help your child to recognize true hunger and satiation
- Make healthy foods taste good and look appealing
- Make meal times at home a fun family event
- Make visits to the fast food outlets a special treat, and not a regular event
- Encourage exercise and outdoor activities
- Limit the time spent with TV and computers
- Keep fast foods and foods high in refined sugars and processed fats out of your pantry

Natural no-calorie-sweeteners such as stevia, xylitol, Nature Sweet Sugar Substitute can be used to partially or fully substitute for added sugar in homemade desserts or soft drinks. These sweeteners do not cause tooth decay.

What healthy snacks can I eat regularly?

- Raw nuts (cashews, Brazils, macadamia, hazelnuts, walnuts, almonds)
- Seeds (sesame seeds, pumpkin seeds, sunflower seeds, hemp seeds, chia seeds, ground flaxseeds, etc) – these

are best stored in the fridge or freezer
- Coconut flesh
- Fresh vegetables - raw and cooked
- Fresh fruits – raw and cooked
- Poultry – free range is best
- All seafood and shellfish (including canned varieties)
- Eggs – the best are free range or organic
- Full fat yoghurt - plain or Greek style, sugar free
- Cheeses - feta, cottage, ricotta, parmesan, romano are good choices
- Red meats such as grass fed lamb, beef or venison
- Cold pressed vegetable, nut and seed oils
- Vinegar – organic apple cider, which encourages weight loss and better digestion
- Avocados and olives
- Spreads made with nuts, hummus, tahini
- Fresh and dried herbs and spices

What unhealthy foods should I avoid?
- Hamburger meat
- Pizza with preserved meats
- Deep-fried foods such as French fries, deep-fried chicken nuggets, fried chicken, deep-fried seafood
- Refined carbohydrates - made with white sugar and white flour
- Sweet fizzy drinks - sodas and diet drinks
- Candies, candies, snack bars, chocolate bars, high in sugar - Dark chocolate is O.K.
- Donuts, croissants, cakes made with refined sugar and white flour
- Processed foods containing hydrogenated vegetable oils
- Margarines containing hydrogenated vegetable oils or trans-fatty acids

- Foods with a lot of pastry such as meat pies and pasties
- Packaged snack foods high in fat, especially hydrogenated oils and trans-fatty acids, such as potato chips, pretzels, corn chips, cookies, packaged muffins and cakes
- Pickled foods with added sugar
- Fruit juices (best to eat the whole fruit)
- In particular it is good to avoid foods that combine high GI carbohydrates with high fat, such as ice cream, pretzels, potato chips, many packaged cakes and biscuits, cream cakes, sweet puddings with custard Foods combining high fat with high GI carbohydrates will cause high insulin levels. The high insulin levels tell our bodies to store fat and not burn fat

Be careful with so called "low fat" snack foods, as we may be inclined to eat twice as much, which will result in more calories than foods with a normal amount of fat.

What are the best non-fattening snacks?

These are to munch when you get unexpectedly hungry and start to crave foods high in sugar, or high GI refined carbohydrates.

Choose from the following selections

- One handful of raw nuts and seeds - these are great for those with Syndrome X because they are low in carbohydrate and are high in fiber and vitamin E
- One handful of raw coconut flesh
- Fresh fruit - 2 pieces maximum at one time
- Fresh crunchy sticks/pieces of celery, carrot, bell peppers, broccoli florets, cherry tomatoes with spicy salsa, or fresh avocado dip, hummus or natural peanut paste
- One small can of crab meat, salmon, sardines or tuna
- A handful of fresh prawns
- Cold roast meat and chicken slices
- Eggs - curried, boiled, poached or made into an omelette with vegetables

- Half an avocado filled with crab meat, or salmon, or tuna
- Plain full fat yogurt (with no added sugar) with fresh fruit (chopped and added by yourself)
- 100 grams (3.5oz) cheese with olives and a chopped apple
- Raw vegetable juices
- Synd-X Protein powder smoothie with fresh berries - use unsweetened milks
- Ryvita cracker with Fetta, Parmesan cheese and/or natural peanut butter

If you feel like a cleansing snack - chop up a mixture of raw vegetables (green beans, lettuce, celery, cucumber, cauliflower, broccoli, bok choy, leeks, sprouts, snow peas, carrots, bell peppers, etc) and serve with a nice dressing poured over using cold pressed oil, squeeze of fresh lemon, Balsamic or apple cider vinegar, garlic and hummus etc.

Satisfying High Fibre Snack Pack -

- ½ cup dried apple or apricots or nectarines, chopped
- 1 cup of almonds, Brazil or macadamia nuts
- ½ cup sunflower seeds
- ¼ cup pumpkin seeds, chopped
- ½ cup hemp seeds
- ½ cup flaked coconut

Mix all together and store in refrigerator - this provides first class protein, fibre and essential fatty acids.

What are the best snacks when eating out?

- BBQ chicken with coleslaw
- BBQ - mixed grill with salad and/or vegetables
- Caesar salad (no croutons)
- Greek salad with fetta cheese and olives
- Roast meat and vegetables
- Steak and vegetables
- Asian foods – choose meat, seafood or tofu and

vegetables. Minimize the rice and noodles
- Chef's salad
- Cauliflower baked with grated Parmesan cheese
- Eggs Florentine
- Steak and eggs or bacon and eggs

What is first class protein?

In nutritional terms when we talk about amino acids, we are referring to the twenty amino acids that are required for the synthesis of proteins in the body. Proteins are large molecules required for the formation of body cells, and they facilitate the chemical reactions in the body that are needed to maintain life.

The twenty amino acids that are needed to manufacture the body's proteins are –

Tyrosine, tryptophan, valine, proline, serine, threonine, lysine, phenylalanine, methionine, glycine, histidine, leucine, isoleucine, cysteine, glutamine, glutamic acid, alanine, aspartic acid, asparagine and arginine.

There are other amino acids present in the body that are not required for protein synthesis, such as taurine and ornithine.

The twenty amino acids that are required to synthesize proteins in the body fall into 2 categories:

- Essential amino acids – there are 8 of these namely - phenylalanine, leucine, isoleucine, threonine, lysine, valine, tryptophan, and methionine. These are classed as essential, as they must be obtained from the diet and cannot be manufactured by the human body.

- Non-essential amino acids – there are 12 of these and they can be made in the body from other compounds.

A protein food is called "First Class" if it contains all of the eight essential amino acids. A first class protein is often referred to as a complete protein.

Examples of first class proteins are:
- Animal meats such as red meat, white meat and poultry
- Seafood
- Eggs
- Dairy products
- Whey protein powder

Foods from the plant kingdom are generally not first class proteins, and these foods need to be combined in specific ways to provide all the eight essential amino acids at one meal.

To derive first class protein from plant foods you need to –

Combine 3 of the following 4 food groups together, at the SAME MEAL –
- Legumes (beans, peas or lentils)
- Grains
- Nuts
- Seeds

So for example, by having a meal containing a grain (rice) with a legume (chickpeas) with a seed (sesame seeds), you will obtain first class protein. By combining a legume (bean) with a grain (barley) and a nut (almonds) you will obtain first class protein.

Many vegetarians do not take enough care in combining their food groups, and protein deficiency is not uncommon in strict vegans. A vegetarian diet lacking in protein can lead to an over reliance on starchy carbohydrates, which may lead to weight gain and fatigue.

Protein is essential for everyone, and especially for people with a weight problem, who need to consume first class protein regularly, at least three times a day. It does not have to be in huge amounts, but should provide all the eight essential amino acids. Complete proteins and pure protein foods either by themselves, or when combined with carbohydrate foods, will moderate the rise in blood glucose and insulin levels after a meal. Indeed eating pure protein with vegetables and no other carbohydrate will usually not cause any significant rise in post-meal blood glucose or insulin levels. This will reduce hunger in between meals and help in the initial stages of weight loss.

What if I am a vegetarian?

To cater for vegetarians many of the recipes in this book are free of animal meats and seafood. You do not have to eat meat, poultry or seafood to follow this eating plan or indeed to overcome insulin resistance; however, many people will find it easier to lose weight if they eat some animal protein.

If you are a strict vegan, you can substitute the meat in the recipes with tofu, tempeh, grains, legumes, nuts and seeds.

As long as you follow our rules for combining at least 3 plant food groups at one meal (as explained before), you will not become deficient in essential amino acids. Strict vegans need to take vitamin B12 supplements daily.

Some people are vegetarian for ethical reasons and this must be respected.

Shopping List for Weight Loss

Beans - there are many varieties such as soybeans, red kidney, pinto, butter, black, adzuki, flageolet, broad, black-eye, Berlotti, cannellini, Garbanzo, etc. The best brands of canned beans and peas are those that have only water and salt added. Baked beans often contain sugar and gluten so avoid this.

Lentils and split peas - red, green, brown and yellow varieties. Lentils should be soaked overnight before cooking. Canned and organic varieties are available.

Chickpeas - dry or canned. They need to be cooked the same way as beans.

Eggs - Free range or organic are best.

Sauces - Miso is fermented bean paste and is made from crushed and boiled soybeans, and is usually mixed with a grain such as rice or barley. Light colored miso is quite sweet whereas the dark and red colored miso is savory. It is important not to boil miso, as it can destroy its nutritional properties. Always add miso at the end of cooking. Miso has a long shelf life - in an airtight container it can last in the refrigerator for one year.

Tamari, soy sauce, oyster sauce, fish sauce, chili sauce, tomato paste.

Noodles - Soba, Rice (flat or round), vermicelli, bean thread noodles and those made with wholegrain ingredients.

Oils - purchase cold pressed oils such as extra virgin olive oil, mustard seed, grape seed, sesame, coconut, walnut and macadamia nut. Store your oils in dark colored bottles, with a tight lid, in a cool dark place. Cold pressed oils are preferable because the oil is extracted from the olive, the seed or nut, by mechanical pressing without the use of solvents or heat, which may damage the oils. Cold pressed oils are much higher in anti-oxidants than are processed oils.

Salt - Celtic, vegetable, herb, rock, sea salt or Gomasio, which is a combination of sesame seeds and rock salt.

Seafood - canned sardines, tuna, trout, crab meat, salmon, mackerel, anchovies and herring. Fresh fish of all varieties such as white fish, blue-fish, sea mullet, sturgeon, trout, southern blue fin tuna, Atlantic and Pacific salmon (fresh), swordfish and squid (calamari) and shell fish of all varieties.

Seaweed - arame, kombu, nori, wakame and kudzu. Seaweed is used extensively in Japanese cuisine. It has many health benefits including its ability to lower cholesterol, and is very high in trace minerals. It is also helpful for those with a sluggish metabolism and underactive thyroid gland problems. Seaweeds are definitely an effective slimming aid.

Nuts and Seeds – pine nuts, walnuts, cashews, macadamias, and Brazil nuts, hazelnuts, almonds, pecans and coconuts. Sunflower seeds, sesame seeds, fresh coconut pieces, pumpkin seeds (pepitas), hempseeds and flaxseed. Nuts and seeds can be ground in a food processor or coffee grinder into a fine powder, which tastes delicious and can be stored in the fridge in an airtight jar. The powder can be added to breakfast cereals or sprinkled over fruit for breakfast. Many people with irritable bowel syndrome and diverticulitis find that they can eat finely groundnuts and seeds without any problems, whereas whole nuts and seeds may aggravate their bowel problems. Nuts and seeds have a very low GI.

Sprouts - bean, snow pea, alfalfa and pea, etc.

Tempeh - some are flavored varieties, also there are many brands that have a combination of tofu and tempeh - found in Super markets, health food stores, and Asian groceries.

Tofu (silken or firm) - found in supermarkets, health food stores and Asian groceries.

Spreads and Dips - Tahini (hulled sesame seed paste), hummus, nut spreads (almond, cashews, Brazil, hazelnuts), natural peanut butter, fresh avocado, olive paste, tomato paste, babaganoush and butter. Spread your bread and crackers with these things instead of margarine.

Vinegar - apple cider, umboshi, rice wine vinegar, white and red wine vinegar. It is worth knowing that ingesting lemon juice or vinegar with food can lower blood glucose levels after eating. You do not have to ingest large amounts of vinegar to achieve this effect. It has been found that only one tablespoon of vinegar in a salad dressing, when eaten with a meal can lower blood glucose levels by up to 30%. Thus it is worthwhile using vinegar or lemon juice regularly with meals. Organic apple cider vinegar is the most beneficial for health of all vinegars. Vinegar, especially apple cider vinegar, can also help to improve weak digestion.

Pasta - whole grain and wheat free brands (if wheat intolerant).

Cereals - oatmeal, rolled oats, wheat germ, cracked wheat, oat or rice bran, pearl barley, whole wheat porridge or gluten free muesli.

Milks – dairy, coconut, oat, almond, soy and rice milk (canned is acceptable). Choose only sugar free varieties.

Mayonnaise - Mayonnaise (with no added sugar).

Breads - pumpernickel, whole grain, stone ground, sprouted wheat bread, whole wheat pita, sourdough, whole grain breads made with cracked wheat, soy, seeds, oats, rye and barley. Choose gluten free if you are gluten intolerant.

Meats - fresh lean beef, veal and pork and lamb.

Poultry - lean fresh chicken, turkey and duck - organic if available.

Vegetables - fresh green leafy of all varieties, salad greens, carrots, beets, sweet potato, new potato, celery, bell peppers, onions, garlic, leeks, shallots, radish, ginger root, parsnip, turnip, pumpkin, bok choy, broccoli, green beans, green peas, Brussels sprouts, cabbage, cauliflower, spinach, artichokes, zucchini, mushrooms, sweet corn, olives, avocado, cucumber, asparagus, eggplant, parsley, coriander, basil and other fresh herbs. Choose many varieties of vegetables with different colors. Roasted peppers and bell peppers, roasted eggplant, marinated vegetables. Tomatoes (fresh and sun dried), tomato puree and tomato paste.

Fermented vegetables are very healthy as they contain trillions of healthy bacteria (probiotics) to help improve the balance of healthy bacteria in your intestines. You can make you own fermented vegetables or buy them in jars premade – a good brand is *Peace Love and Veggies* made by an Australian company in Byron Bay

Asian vegetables - Galangal tastes like sour ginger, and also similar in looks to ginger. Peel and slice, as you would ginger. Often found in Thai, Malaysian and Indonesian dishes. Has a similar uplifting affect like ginger.

Shiitake Mushrooms these Japanese mushrooms are available either fresh (used within a day or two), or dried (can be kept indefinitely in a jar). The fresh mushrooms are firm and dry unlike the field mushroom, which is quite moist. The stems are too tough to eat but are great to use for flavor in stocks. To prepare the dried mushrooms, soak in warm water for 30 minutes, remove the stalks, strain and use the liquid for stocks or soups. To prepare fresh mushrooms, wipe the cap, remove the stalks and use according to the recipe. They are a great source of potassium and fiber and are beneficial for the immune system. Exotic mushrooms can be bought from either Asian grocers or health food stores and some green grocers.

Spices - chili (powder, paste or fresh), black peppercorns, mustard (Dijon and whole seed), ground cumin, paprika, basil, cloves, coriander, turmeric, garlic (fresh or paste), curry powder and curry pastes.

Fruits - best to choose those in season - all citrus fruits, cherries, plums, apples, bananas, pears, peaches, apricots, grapes, mango, figs, nectarines, berries of all varieties, water melon, honeydew melon, and custard apples. Indeed all fruits are beneficial to health.

Toasting Seeds and Nuts

The easiest method for most seeds (such as sesame and caraway), and pine nuts is to pre-heat a fry pan, add a small amount of oil, sprinkle the seeds or nuts in the pan and gently turn with a wooden spoon until lightly toasted. Watch them carefully as they can burn very quickly. Remove them from the fry pan and place on absorbent paper to cool.

Almonds and other nuts can be dry roasted over moderate heat in a pan, or on a tray in a moderate oven, or if you wish, use the same method as for the seeds.

If prepared in advance the toasted nuts or seeds can be stored in an airtight container in your pantry or kitchen cupboard. Remember to eat plenty of your nuts raw (un-roasted) as they are very healthy when raw.

Preparing Legumes

Legumes consist of beans, peas and lentils. Many varieties are now available in cans and only need to be rinsed and drained before being combined with other ingredients.

You can prepare dry uncooked legumes with the following method -

- Soak the legumes in a saucepan with two to three times their volume of cold water. It is often most convenient to soak them overnight.
- Drain the water, rinse the beans, and add new water using three times the amount of water as the beans.
- Bring the water to the boil and simmer the beans until they are tender.
- Drain the water off.

Cooking times will vary according to the size and type of the legume. Legumes are cooked when they are just soft when you squeeze them.

Do not overcook the legumes or they will become "mushy" and are then unsuitable for salads. If overcooked they can be used in soups or casseroles. You can freeze any leftover legumes in an airtight freezer bag, draw as much air from the bag as you can, seal and freeze.

You can also store cooked beans in an airtight container for several days in the fridge.

The GI of cooked beans is generally lower than that of canned beans; however it is acceptable to use canned beans for convenience, as long as they do not contain added sugar.

Balancing the Food Groups for Weight Control

The maintenance eating plan in this book is designed to provide an approximate total calorie breakdown as follows -

- 40 to 45% from low GI carbohydrates, largely from vegetables and fruits
- 25 to 30% from healthy fats
- 25 to 30% from first class lean protein

These percentages are approximations and can be varied but do not increase the amount of carbohydrate. It is safer to increase the amount of healthy fats and protein.

If you feel that you desire to eat a meal with more fat, then choose the healthy fats from eggs, cold pressed oils, seafood, cheese, avocados and nuts. Avoid deep fried foods.

Let's look at a few examples to see how the theory works. If you are eating a total of 2,000 calories daily here is a possible breakdown of food groups -

Percentage	Daily Calories	Food Group
100%	2000	all groups
40% C	800	200 grams carbohydrate (4 calories per gram)
30% F	600	67 grams fat (9 calories per gram)
30% P	600	150 grams protein (4 calories per gram)

Foot Note: Carbohydrates = C, Protein = P, Fat = F

As another example, if you are eating a total of 1200 calories daily here is a possible breakdown of food groups –

Percentage	Daily Calories	Food Group
100%	1200	all groups
40% C	480	120 grams carbohydrate (4 calories per gram)
30% F	360	40 grams fat (9 calories per gram)
30% P	360	90 grams protein (4 calories per gram)

Foot Note: Carbohydrates = C, Protein = P, Fat = F

Are you metabolically resistant ?

There are some people who are extremely resistant to losing weight even though they may have spent a life time dieting. They have often tried every possible diet including low-fat low-calorie diets (such as the HCG Diet) with only a total calorie content of 500 calories per day. Many of them have given up in desperation after a lifetime of being a yo-yo dieter. Many of these metabolically resistant people are overly sensitive to "normal" or conventionally accepted healthy amounts of carbohydrate. They find that they are unable to lose weight unless they follow a ketogenic diet where the amount of carbohydrate consumed daily is only around 20 grams.

How to kick-start a very slow metabolism

To enable weight loss to begin we must kick-start the metabolism in these difficult metabolically resistant patients. This means a very low carbohydrate diet along the lines of the ketogenic diet. Some popular high-protein high-fat diets allow as little as 6 to 18% of daily calories to be obtained from carbohydrate. There is no doubt that this strategy can work for these very resistant patients. It can be very effective to initially reduce the dietary carbohydrate intake to these extremely low levels. This can allow weight loss to begin.

Let's look at 2 examples of extremely low carbohydrate diets -

Let us say you are eating 1200 calories a day with only 10% of these calories being provided by carbohydrate foods

Percentage	Daily Calories	Food Group
100%	1200	all groups
10% C	120	30 grams carbohydrate (4 calories per gram)
45% F	540	60 grams fat (9 calories per gram)
45% P	540	135 grams protein (4 calories per gram)

Foot Note: Carbohydrates = C, Protein = P, Fat = F

Let us say you are eating 1200 calories a day with only 6% of these calories being provided by carbohydrate foods.

Percentage	Daily Calories	Food Group
100%	1200	all groups
6% C	72	18 grams carbohydrate (4 calories per gram)
47% F	564	62.7 grams fat (9 calories per gram)
47% P	564	141 grams protein (4 calories per gram)

Foot Note: Carbohydrates = C, Protein = P, Fat = F

Ketosis

In those who are fasting or following a very low carbohydrate diet (less than 40 grams per day), the metabolic state of ketosis may occur in the body. Some people will need to consume less than 20grams of carbohydrate per day to enable ketosis to begin. In the state of ketosis your body will be burning its stored fat for energy instead of carbohydrates. You should not feel hungry which is in contrast to people on a low-fat high-carbohydrate diet.

Ketosis is recognizable because there are measurable levels of ketones in the blood, urine, stools and the breath. It is possible to use urine test strips (Ketostix), which test for the presence of ketones in the urine. The Ketostix result gives you an indication of the amount of ketones you are excreting from your body, and thus your degree of fat burning (lipolysis). If there are ketones present in the urine, the test strips turn a pink to purple color, depending upon the amount of ketones present. The more ketones present in the urine, the darker will be the purple color.

Interpreting the results of Ketostix

Color	Meaning
Pink (1.5 or small)	You are burning fat gradually
Purple (4 to 16)	You are burning fat quickly
Trace (negative)	You are eating too many carbohydrates to be in ketosis

The test strips are available under the brand name of Keto-stix.

Do the urine testing twice daily. The end of the Ketostix strip is placed into a mid-steam specimen of urine, after it has been collected in a jar. If you are following an extremely low carbohydrate diet (less than 20 grams per day), you will show ketones in your urine indicating that you are burning fat. Generally speaking you will have enough carbohydrate stored as glycogen in your body for only 48 hours, and after you have used it all up, you will enter a state of ketosis.

If your urine strips do not turn pink to purple on a low carbohydrate diet, this is nothing to worry about. As long as you are losing weight and feeling well, the program in this book is still working efficiently. This means that you are still burning fat and producing ketones, but only small quantities of ketones, which are insufficient to cause a color change on the test strips.

Cautions for ketogenic diets

If you decide to go on a very low carbohydrate diet (less than 40 grams of carbohydrate per day), you MUST do this under the supervision of your own doctor and/or naturopath. This applies to everyone and especially to those who are obese (with a body mass index of over 30), those with medical problems such as heart disease, kidney disease, or any other chronic medical problem. You will need to drink at least 80 to 90 ounces (2.5 liters) of water daily while in the state of ketosis.

When first entering the state of ketosis you may experience unpleasant symptoms due to detoxification and mild metabolic acidosis. These may include headaches, nausea, fatigue or dizziness. In those with a tendency to gout, a ketogenic diet may increase the risk of an acute attack of gouty arthritis. This is because the blood uric acid levels increase, as the uric acid competes with ketones for excretion in the urine. High uric acid levels increase the risk of kidney problems, so those with impaired kidney function should not follow a ketogenic diet unless it is recommended and supervised by their own doctor.

Drinking plenty of water and taking a liver tonic powder such as LivaTone will reduce the detoxification symptoms of a ketogenic diet.

Insulin dependent diabetics are not able to follow a ketogenic diet (extremely low carbohydrate diet) unless their own doctor advises it. This is because it can lead to metabolic problems, which may destabilize their blood glucose control and lead to dangerous metabolic problems.

The Ketogenic Diet

The Ketogenic Diet provides extremely low amounts of carbohydrate (less than 20 grams daily) which force your body into a state of ketosis and quick fat burning. The Ketogenic Diet is very effective at initializing weight loss in metabolically resistant patients.

These extremely low carbohydrate diets are best followed under the supervision of a health care professional, and are not practical to accept as a way of life for long periods of time. You can see from the tables earlier, that when the carbohydrate intake is drastically reduced, it is necessary to greatly increase the amount of fat and protein in the diet to meet calorie requirements. If these very large amounts of protein and/or fat are consumed for long periods, you will need to be supervised by your health care professional as metabolic problems such as high uric acid levels and constipation may occur. When you are on these extremely low carbohydrate diets, you will need to eat large amounts of green leafy vegetables and salad greens to support your kidney and liver function and to avoid becoming too acidic and to avoid constipation.

Ketostix

The use of the Ketostix urine testing strips can be helpful when you are trying to determine the maximum daily amount of carbohydrate that you can eat, before you bust out of the fat burning zone.

You need to find the daily amount of carbohydrate that will keep the Ketostix testing in the purple color range, which indicates that you are in the fat burning zone. While in the fat burning zone you will be eliminating enough ketones in the urine to make the Ketostix turn purple. If you eat too much carbohydrate your metabolism will shift out of the fat burning zone into the carbohydrate burning zone, and the excretion of ketones in the urine will fall to lower levels which are insufficient to turn the Ketostix purple. To lose weight quickly you need to keep the ketostix purple.

Everyone has an individual metabolism, but generally less than 20g of carbohydrate daily, will keep you well and truly in the fat burning and ketone-producing zone. Some people may find that they can eat more than 20g of carbohydrate daily, and still stay in the fat burning zone with purple Ketostix. This takes some trial and error but eventually you will find the maximum daily intake of carbohydrate that allows you to stay in the fat burning zone of ketosis with purple Ketostix. You can use the carbohydrate counter on page 322 to help you work this out.

Use of Ketostix urine testing strips

Amount of Ketones in urine	Color Change
Negative (no ketones)	very light pink
Trace = 0.5mmol/L	light pink
Small = 1.5mmol/L	bright pink
Moderate = 4mmol/L	purple
Large = 8mmol/L	dark purple
Very large = 16mmol/L	very dark purple

There is a color code on the Ketostix container to compare your testing strips with to determine the amount of ketones in your urine. The directions on the container must be followed exactly to get an accurate measurement. Ketostix testing strips can be purchased from your local pharmacy.

A SAMPLE KETOGENIC DIET

Breakfast

2	*large whole eggs*
½ oz (15gm)	*bacon, with fat*
2 tbsp	*butter*
1 oz (28 gm)	*spinach*
½ oz (15gm)	*tomatoes*

Calories 521 Carbs 4 to 5gms

Lunch

3 oz (85 gm)	*chicken breast slices, skin on*
2 tbsp	*olive oil*
1	*lime or lemon*
2	*celery stalks*
2 ½ cups	*mixed greens*

Calories 800 Carbs 9gms

Dinner

4 oz (115gm)	*rump steak, grilled*
1 cup	*mushrooms, chopped*
2 tbsp	*cream*
1 cup	*string beans or broccoli florets*
2 tbsp	*butter*

Calories 650 Carbs 8gms

Extra points for slimming

Also remember it is not only how much you eat that's important, but rather what you eat that will cause the chemical and hormonal imbalances that lead to weight excess. The real enemy is refined carbohydrate, and especially sugar, which will send your insulin levels sky rocketing. I well remember a well-known naturopath in Adelaide South Australia, who used to tell his patients that white sugar should be called "white death".

If you are hungry please eat enough to satisfy your own natural hunger. Your appetite will vary according to the amount of exercise you do, and also according to your body weight. So if you need food, eat healthy food choices from our Syndrome X Shopping List.

Our recipes provide plenty of raw fruits and vegetables to provide antioxidants and cancer fighting phyto-nutrients. Raw foods are essential to improve your liver function and cleanse the lymphatic system, and some raw vegetables and/ or fruits should be eaten with EVERY meal.

The meals largely composed of seafood, meat, poultry, eggs or cheese are higher in protein and lower in carbohydrates than meals based upon vegetables and legumes.

Features of Insulin Resistance

Abnormalities in blood fats

Cholesterol

Elevated insulin levels stimulate your liver to produce excess amounts of the unhealthy LDL cholesterol. In those with Syndrome X there may be low levels of the good HDL cholesterol, and excessively high levels of the bad LDL cholesterol. If the LDL cholesterol becomes damaged by the high sugar levels in the blood, it can cause a lot of inflammation.

Normal levels of HDL cholesterol are (38 to 72 mg/dL) in men and (46 to 87 mg/dL) in women.

Normal levels of LDL cholesterol are (19 to 133 mg/dL).

Triglycerides

Triglycerides are lightweight small fatty particles that have only a very small amount of protein attached to them. Most of the triglycerides are stored as fat in your fat deposits. The triglyceride fats are manufactured in the liver, which converts them to very low-density lipoproteins abbreviated to VLDL. High levels of triglycerides and VLDL will not only increase weight gain, they will increase your risk of cardiovascular disease.

Today many people have become obsessed with cholesterol and think it is the main predictor of heart disease. Indeed many overweight people never bother to take note of their triglyceride levels in their blood tests. High triglyceride levels by themselves, irrespective of cholesterol levels, are a potent risk factor for heart disease. Indeed high triglyceride levels are just as important as smoking, obesity and high blood pressure in increasing your chances of heart disease. High triglycerides make your blood thick and sticky so that it does not flow freely around inside your blood vessels - this increases the risk of blood clots and this equals a higher chance of strokes and heart attacks.

Normal triglyceride levels are 0.1 to 2.0mmol/L or 9 to 177mg/dL, and the lower they are within this normal range, the better off you are.

Make sure that you are fasting (do not eat/drink anything but water for 12 to 14 hours before the blood test), when you have your blood taken to measure the triglyceride levels. This is because triglyceride levels can be temporarily much higher just after eating.

It is relieving to know that changing what you eat, exercising a little and taking some supplements is able to reverse this deadly combination within a few months, and sometimes sooner. And you will not have to follow a low-fat, low-calorie diet to do this, so you will not be hungry or miserable. A study at Harvard University in 1966, showed that very high triglyceride levels could be reduced greatly with a very low carbohydrate diet *(REF. 3)*

A diet high in refined carbohydrates and low in protein and fat, will increase insulin, which will cause an elevation in the triglyceride levels. *(REF. 4)*

Abnormalities in glucose levels

In those with Syndrome X the blood glucose levels are often unstable, and can vary from too low to too high. Over time the blood glucose levels generally become too high. Syndrome X can eventually lead to type 2 diabetes because the insulin resistance gets worse, causing blood glucose levels to rise.

Hypoglycemia (very low blood sugar levels)

When the blood glucose levels drop below 2.5 to 3 mmol/L (45 to 54 mg/dL), the following symptoms may occur -

- Strong cravings for sugar or alcohol

- Imbalances in brain function leading to anxiety, poor concentration, foggy brain, poor memory, irritability, depression and headaches
- Sleep disturbances, such as waking suddenly from sleep with anxiety and palpitations, bad dreams, and restless sleep
- Mental and physical fatigue which can be overwhelming and tends to occur in between meals and especially in the mid afternoon

Hypoglycemic symptoms can be devastating, and it is not uncommon to find sufferers who think they are battling with a mental illness. Antidepressant drugs will not help these symptoms, as they do not correct the underlying unstable blood glucose levels. Many people with depression and addictions can be helped with an eating program and supplements to stabilize their blood glucose levels. The sugar addiction can become so strong that you feel totally out of control until you can get your sugar hit.

How is insulin resistance diagnosed?

Your own doctor may be interested in doing laboratory tests to see if you have Syndrome X.

You will need to have your blood taken in the fasting state, which means that you should not eat/drink anything apart from pure water, for 12 hours before the blood is taken. It is easiest to fast overnight and have your blood taken before breakfast.

Fasting Blood Glucose Level (BGL)

If your fasting BGL is over 6.1 mmol/L (110mg/dL), this means that insulin is starting to lose control over your glucose metabolism. This is a sign of insulin resistance.

Glucose Tolerance Test

The Glucose Tolerance Test (GTT) measures the tolerance of an individual for a load of administered glucose. If your tolerance for this extra load of glucose is normal, then your blood levels of glucose will remain within the normal range. If your tolerance for this extra load of glucose is impaired, your blood glucose levels will become higher than the normal range (see table 1).

If you have impaired glucose tolerance, this will be because you have insulin resistance, meaning that your insulin is incapable of controlling your blood glucose levels. If your blood glucose levels become even higher you will be classed as a diabetic, which could be due to severe insulin resistance or insulin failure.

The GTT will only be accurate if you follow a relatively high carbohydrate diet (200 grams daily) for four days before the test.

The GTT measures your blood glucose (glucose) levels after you ingest a test dose of glucose. The blood glucose levels are measured over a period of several hours, depending on whether the doctor has ordered a 2-hour GTT, or a 3-hour GTT which goes for longer.

You may be asked to fill out a questionnaire of your symptoms during the period of the GTT, with the aim of matching your symptoms to the reading of your blood glucose level. Symptoms such as faintness, shaking, sweating, palpitations, nausea, mood changes, mental confusion, headaches and extreme hunger are suggestive of very low blood glucose levels, or an abnormally rapid drop in the blood glucose levels. Even if you are not asked to fill out a questionnaire, it is a good idea to keep a record of your symptoms and their timing during the GTT. This may help your doctor to interpret the significance of your blood glucose levels, to the way you feel day to day.

Subtle abnormalities in the GTT often occur in those with Syndrome X, a long time before the onset of diabetes.

Blood Sugar Levels during GTT

Time	Normal Levels	Impaired Glucose Tolerance	Diabetes
Fasting	3.6 to 6.1 *mmol/L* (65 to 110 mg/dL)	6.1 to 6.9 *mmol/L* (113 to 124 mg/dL)	over 6.9 *mmol/L* (over 124 mg/dL)
2 hour	Less than 7.1 *mmol/L* (Less than 128 mg/dL)	7.2 to 11.0 *mmol/L* (130 to 198 mg/dL)	over 11 *mmol/L* (over 198 mg/dL)

Table 1

The one-hour blood glucose level is not always reported, but generally speaking a level over 9.0 mmol/L (162 mg/dL) is considered abnormal, and is indicative of impaired glucose tolerance.

Ideally insulin levels should be tested along with the blood glucose levels during the GTT. The accepted normal value for the 2-hour level of insulin varies between the experts. According to some experts the 2-hour insulin level is abnormally elevated if it is above 1.5 times your age, up to the age of 50. Using this method a 2-hour insulin level over 75 would be abnormally high for any person.

Serum Insulin Levels

It is worthwhile to measure insulin levels, as it is the high insulin levels caused by insulin resistance, which is the cause of Syndrome X.

A laboratory accustomed to measuring insulin levels should do the testing of your insulin levels. The specimen of blood should be frozen and the test must be completed within 24 hours of taking the blood. If these procedures are not followed the results may be inaccurate.

Excessive blood levels of insulin (hyperinsulinemia) are diagnosed by finding an elevated fasting blood insulin level, or by finding elevated insulin two hours after giving the patient a 75 gram dose of pure glucose.

Many research laboratories use the fasting normal levels of insulin in healthy young people as the standard reference against which we measure a patient's blood insulin levels. Generally speaking if your fasting insulin level is over 12 mU/L, you probably have some degree of Syndrome X. The greater your insulin level is over 12, the greater your insulin resistance is. If we use 12 as the upper limit of normal for fasting insulin levels, a result of 36 would mean that it requires 3 times the normal amount of insulin to keep your blood glucose levels at their current value. Some laboratories will set the upper limit of normal fasting insulin levels as high as 20, but this will miss some people with insulin resistance.

Normal insulin levels during a GTT are considered to be the following:

Time	Normal Serum Insulin (in mU/L)
Fasting	less than 12 (some labs will report anything below 20 as normal)
1 hour	9 to 75
2 hour	5 to 50
3 hour	1 to 24

Table 2

Some laboratories have different "normal ranges" for serum insulin, which are higher than the above values, and may miss some people with Syndrome X. For example some laboratories will state that insulin levels below 76 are normal, while insulin levels above 80 indicate insulin resistance. They qualify this by saying that insulin levels between 75 to 80 are in a "grey area" and may indicate insulin resistance. I think the lower levels in table 2 are more realistic, and if used for evaluation, will not miss as many people who are in the early stages of Syndrome X. See graph on page 24.

Glycosylated hemoglobin levels

The blood test called Glycosylated Hemoglobin (often abbreviated to HbA1c, Hgb A1, or GHB) is very useful. The measurement of HbA1c levels evaluates the amount of glucose that has been present in your blood over the previous 3 months. The lower your level of HbA1c is, the better you will be, as far as blood glucose control is concerned. The normal laboratory range for HbA1c is (4 to 6%).

Blood fats

Fats	Normal range (in mmol/L)	Normal range (in mg/dL)
Total cholesterol	3.9 to 5.5	148 to 209
Triglycerides	0.1 to 2.0	9 to 177
LDL cholesterol	0.5 to 3.5	19 to 133
HDL cholesterol male	1.0 to 1.9	38 to 72
HDL cholesterol female	1.2 to 2.3	46 to 87

Cholesterol/HDL ratio	Risk Of Heart Disease
1. to 3.5	below average (desirable)
2. to 5.5	average
5.6 to 8.3	high > 8.3 very high

Liver Function tests

It is not uncommon to find that the blood levels of liver enzymes are slightly elevated in those with Syndrome X, especially if they are carrying excess weight in the abdominal area. This is usually associated with some degree of fatty liver. The infiltration of unhealthy fat into the liver causes some inflammation of the liver cells. Liver enzymes become elevated when the liver is inflamed.

LIVER TESTS	NORMAL RANGES
Total Bilirubin	0.18 to 1.0 mg/dL
Liver Enzymes	
AST	5 to 45 U/L
ALT	5 to 45 U/L
AP	30 to 120 U/L
GT	5 to 35 U/L

Sex hormone levels

In women, high levels of insulin tend to increase the blood levels of the male hormone testosterone, and reduce the levels of the protein called Sex Hormone Binding Globulin (SHBG). This results in raised levels of the free testosterone in the blood. The free testosterone is unbound to the SHBG, and is far more active than testosterone which is bound up.

In women, high levels of free testosterone increase the tendency to gain excess fat in the upper part of the body and the abdomen.

Elevated male hormones may cause facial hair, acne and/or male pattern balding. Hormone treatments include natural progesterone cream or the anti-male hormone medication called Cyproterone Acetate. These hormone treatments are very effective in overcoming these problems, and may also help with weight loss.

The normal range for free androgens is measured as the Free Androgen Index (FAI) and is:

Sex	FAI normal range
Males	40 to 170
Females	0.1 to 7

Note: The word androgen means male hormone.

Glycemic Index of Foods

The Glycemic Index (GI) measures the effect of a specific food upon your blood glucose levels after you eat it.

The standard against which all foods are measured on the Glycemic Index (GI) scale is pure glucose, which is given a GI rating of 100. Every other food is measured on a scale from 0 to 100 depending upon its effect on blood glucose levels.

Different types of carbohydrate foods will have very different effects upon your blood glucose levels and therefore your insulin levels. Carbohydrates cause blood glucose and insulin levels to rise more rapidly than any other types of foods. This applies especially to refined carbohydrates, which are digested and rapidly absorbed from the gut into the blood stream. However if a carbohydrate food is absorbed slowly from the gut, less insulin is required. It is not just the amount of carbohydrate you eat that's important, it's the type of carbohydrate you eat that also determines the magnitude of the rise in blood glucose levels.

Food	Carbohydrate (g)	Calories	GI
Honey 1 tbsp	17g	68	58
Lima beans ½ cup	17g	68	32

From the above you can see that 1 tbsp honey = ½ cup Lima beans = 17grams carbohydrate = 68 calories. So you may ask which is likely to be the most fattening food? Well they contain the same amount of carbohydrate and thus the same amount of calories, so they should be equally fattening - right?

Well this is not necessarily right!

The higher GI of the honey means that 1 tbsp of honey will raise your blood glucose more than ½ cup of Lima beans. This may not matter in those who are not overweight and do not suffer with Syndrome X. However those with Syndrome X will find that the 1 tbsp of honey is more fattening than the ½ cup of Lima beans because the honey causes their blood glucose to rise more. This means that they will pump out more insulin, and we all know that insulin promotes the conversion of glucose into fat. So we are not just talking about grams of carbohydrate and number of calories, we are talking about the metabolic effect of a specific type of carbohydrate food in your body - that is what the GI is all about. As they say "one calorie is not always equal to one calorie" when it comes to your weight!

This may seem confusing but the bottom line is -

• If you are trying to choose between 2 foods that have equivalent amounts of carbohydrates - choose the one with the lower GI.
• Foods that have a high GI raise your blood glucose levels higher and faster than foods that have a low GI.
• For people with Syndrome X, obesity or type 2 diabetes, it is far better to choose foods that have a low GI.

Low GI foods are desirable because -

• They do not cause the blood glucose levels to rise rapidly
• They prevent high insulin levels and therefore the storage of fat
• They are more filling and reduce hunger

It has been shown that lowering the Glycemic Index (GI) of the carbohydrates ingested (without changing the total amount of carbohydrate) improves blood glucose control by 10%.

The Glycemic Index (GI) of foods is now internationally recognized as being important in healthy food choices. The World Health Organization (WHO) now recommends that people should choose foods that have a low GI.

You will find low GI carbohydrate in foods such as legumes (beans, dried peas, lentils), whole gains such as oats, wheat, spelt, amaranth, quinoa, barley, millet, brown rice, vegetables (except for white potatoes) and many fruits. Tart tasting fruits (such as citrus, passion fruit, kiwi) have a lower GI.

Gluten containing grains, even if they are low GI, may cause weight problems in some people – see page 204

Vegetable carbohydrates

Higher carbohydrate vegetables are potato, sweet potato, carrots, pumpkin and corn; although corn and sweet potato are lower than potatoes. Beet and peas contain carbohydrates; however normal serving sizes do not have a significant effect upon blood glucose levels. If starchy vegetables such as carrots, pumpkin and potatoes are eaten in normal serving sizes accompanied by protein, they will not cause significant problems for those trying to lose weight. However you will find it easier to lose weight if you avoid the starchy vegetables during the first 8 weeks of the eating plan in this book - see page 34.

Vegetables used for salads such as celery, tomatoes, cucumber, zucchini, leafy greens, lettuce, snow peas, onion, garlic, bell peppers, etc. contain very slowly digested carbohydrates and you can eat them freely.

Swap high-GI foods for low-GI foods

Here are some ideas to help you swap from undesirable high GI foods to desirable low GI foods

High GI Foods	Low GI Food Substitutes
Packaged snack foods such as chips, pretzels, cakes, muffins bagels, candies, lollies and cookies. Dried fruits.	Fresh whole fruits, nuts and seeds. Ryvita crackers. Plain full fat yogurt. Roasted legumes. Avocado. Olives. Cheeses.

High GI Foods	Low GI Food Substitutes
White Rice (instant) Pastas made with refined flour	Long grain rice, brown rice, wild rice, basmati rice, lentils, beans and chickpeas
Potato	Legumes, sweet potatoes,
Processed breakfast cereals	Raw muesli made from oats, nuts, seeds (hemp, chia, sunflower etc), LSA and psyllium.
Breads especially white, but also some types of processed whole wheat bread containing sugar	Pumpernickel or breads made with hemp, almond, coconut, soy or baisen flour
Savory biscuits (crackers) such as Salada, jatz, rice crackers	Ryvita, Corn and rice thins

The GI scale applies to carbohydrate foods. Foods mainly comprised of fat and/or protein do not raise the blood glucose levels significantly.

Some low GI carbohydrates

Bread

Chapati is flat Indian bread. The best type with the lowest GI of only 27 is made from chickpea flour (also known as baisen flour). Pumpernickel has a low GI of 51 and Sourdough bread has a low GI of 52. Stone ground breads such as whole-wheat stone-ground bread, have a low GI of 53. In stone ground breads the entire grain is used and is a rich source of fiber, B vitamins and zinc.

Cereals

Oat bran and oatmeal of the old fashioned type (not instant) have a low GI of around 50. Pearl barley has a very low GI of only 25. Pearl barley can be used as a breakfast cereal or in place of rice, and also added to soups or casseroles.

Bulgur is cracked wheat and has a GI of 48. Bulgur is used in "tabouli", which is a salad combination of onion, tomato, parsley and bulgur. Bulgur can also be used in vegetarian burgers, stews and casseroles or as a low GI cereal. Rice bran has a very low GI of only 19. Rice bran can be added to breakfast cereals, muffins and cookies. The GI of rice varies a lot depending upon the type of rice. The low GI varieties of rice are brown, Basmati and Japonica. Waxy or glutinous rice and Arborio rice have a higher GI.

Legumes

Beans of all varieties, lentils and chickpeas are generally low GI carbohydrates. In Asia soft blended lentils known as dhal (pronounced daal), provide a healthy low GI carbohydrate accompaniment to a meal.

Fruits

Apples are high in fiber and provide a low GI snack. The GI of a fresh raw apple is only 38. Apples contain a lot of fructose (fruit sugar), which is more slowly absorbed than glucose and has a low GI of 23.

Oranges have a low GI of 44, are full of vitamin C, and make an excellent snack. Fresh grapefruit has a low GI of only 25 and can be eaten with other fruits, or sprinkled with stevia or Nature Sweet Sugar Substitute to temper their tart taste. Fresh peaches have a low GI of 42 and make an excellent high fiber snack.

Fresh pears are high in fructose, which does not cause blood glucose to rise significantly. Pears are good for a snack, with breakfast or for dessert and when fresh and raw their GI is only 38.

Fresh cherries are an excellent fruit for those with Syndrome X, as they have the lowest GI of any fruit. Cherries can be used widely and have a low GI index of only 22. Plums are very nutritious with a low GI of 39. Green Grapes are quite high in fruit acids and have a GI of 46. They make a convenient snack especially with raw nuts. Of all the tropical fruits, kiwi, mango and papaya have the lowest GI of between 50 and 60.

Carbohydrate Counter

Grams of Carbohydrate in foods

Vegetables	Carbohydrates (g)
Alfalfa sprouts 100g	3
Artichoke 1 medium	12
Asparagus 4 spears	2.2
Avocado peeled 50g	3.5
Bamboo shoots 1 cup canned	4
Bean sprouts 100g	3
Beans-green 1 cup cooked	6.8
Beans-green 25g	2
Beets ½ cup cooked	8.5
Bell peppers 40g	2
Broccoli 1 cup cooked	8.5
Broccoli 50g	3
Brussels sprouts cooked 100g	4
Cabbage 1 cup cooked	6.2
Cabbage cooked 30g	1.5
Carrots ½ cup cooked	8.2
Carrots 100g	4
Cauliflower ½ cup cooked	2.9
Cauliflower cooked 50g	2.5
Celery 1 stalk	1.6
Chives raw 2 tbsp	1
Coleslaw 1 cup	8.5
Collard greens 1 cup	5
Corn sweet ½ cup cooked	20.6
Cucumber 1cup sliced raw	3.6

Vegetables	Carbohydrates (g)
Dandelion 1 cup	6.7
Eggplant ½ cup cooked	3.2
Endive 1 cup	2.1
Frozen vegetables 1 cup	24
Garlic 1 clove	1
Ginger ¼ cup raw	3
Kale ½ cup cooked	6.7
Kohlrabi 1 cup cooked	8.7
Leeks ½ cup cooked	4
Lettuce 1 leaf	0.4
Mushrooms 1 cup	3.1
Mustard greens 1 cup cooked	5.6
New potato 1 small	28
Onion 1 tbsp	0.9
Parsley 1 tbsp	0.3
Parsnips 1 cup cooked	23
Peas-green 1 cup cooked	19.4
Peas-green 1 cup frozen	23
Pepper or bell peppers 1 cup raw	7
Potato 1 baked	33
Potato salad 1 cup	33.5
Pumpkin 1 cup cooked	20
Radish 4 fresh	1
Spinach ½ cup cooked	3.4
Summer squash 1 cup cooked	8
Sweet potato 1 baked	37
Tomato 1 small	5
Turnips 1 cup cooked	11.3
Water chestnuts canned 1 cup	17

Vegetables	Carbohydrates (g)
Winter squash 1 cup cooked	18
Zucchini 1 cup cooked	8

Fruits - fresh & raw	Carbohydrates (g)
Apple 1 medium	20
Apricots 1	4.6
Apricots dried 5 to 6 pieces	2.6
Avocado 1 medium	20
Banana 1	26.6
Blackberries ½ cup	9.2
Blueberries ½ cup	11
Cantaloupe ½ small	22
Cherries ½ cup	10.2
Dates 5	27
Figs 50g	22
Grapefruit pink ½	10.3
Grapefruit yellow ½	5
Grapes green 100g	15
Honey dew melon ½ cup	7.2
Kiwi 1 medium	9
Lemon 1	6
Lemon juice 1 cup	21
Mango 1	35
Nectarine 1	16
Olives 4	trace
Orange 1	16
Papaya 1 medium	30.4
Peach 1 large	10
Peach dried 1 cup	48

Fruits - fresh & raw	Carbohydrates (g)
Peaches canned ½ cup	19
Pear 1	21
Pineapple 1 cup fresh	21.2
Pineapple 2 slices fresh	10
Pineapple canned 1 cup	52
Plum 1 medium	9
Prune 1	5.6
Raisins 40g	28
Raspberries 1 cup	14
Raspberries ½ cup	10.5
Red & green grapes ⅓ cup	7.9
Rhubarb 1 cup	7.5
Strawberries ½ cup	5.3
Tomato ½ cup	2.9
Tomato juice 1 cup	10.4
Watermelon 1 cup	8

Legumes cooked	Carbohydrates (g)
Baked beans canned ½ cup	24
Black beans ¾ cup	31
Black-eyed peas 1 cup	38
Chana dal 1½ cups	28
Chickpeas boiled ½ cup	23
Chickpeas canned ½ cup	30
Lentils ½ cup	18
Lima beans 1 cup	33.7
Navybeans 1 cup	40.3
Pinto beans ½ cup	20
Pinto beans canned ½ cup	25

Legumes cooked	Carbohydrates (g)
Red kidney beans boiled ½ cup	20
Red kidney beans canned ½ cup	25
Soy milk unsweetened 1 cup	13
Soybeans ½ cup	10
Split peas ½ cup	20
Tofu frozen dessert 60g	21
Tofu/bean curd 2-inch cube	2.9

Nuts and Seeds	Carbohydrates (g)
Almond paste 30g	14.5
Almonds 30g	6
Brazil 30g	3.1
Cashews 60g	18
Coconut flesh 30g	4.3
Coconut milk canned 100g	4
Hazelnuts 30g	4.7
Macadamia 60g	10
Peanut butter natural 1 tbsp	3
Peanuts 30g	5.4
Pecans 30g	4.1
Pistachio 60g	14
Pumpkin seeds 30g	4.2
Sesame 1 tbsp 1.4 Walnuts 30g	4.2
Sunflower seeds 30g	5.6

Dairy (Cow's Milk) Products	Carbohydrates (g)
Camembert 30g	0.5
Cheddar Cheese 30g	1
Chocolate milk 1 cup	26

Dairy (Cow's Milk) Products	Carbohydrates (g)
Cottage skim 1 cup	10
Cottage whole 1 cup	7
Cream light 1 tbsp	1
Cream sour 1 tbsp	0.5
Cream thick 1 tbsp	0.5
Cream whipped 2 tbsp	1
Feta 30g	1
Ice cream ½ cup	15
Ricotta skim 1 cup	13
Ricotta whole milk 1 cup	7
Skim milk 1 cup	12
Swiss 30g	1
Whole milk 1 cup	11
Yogurt fruit low fat 1 cup	43
Yogurt plain skim 1 cup	13
Yogurt plain whole 1 cup	12

Grains and Cereals	Carbohydrates (g)
All bran ½ cup	22
Barley ½ cup - cooked	35
Buckwheat ½ cup - cooked	20
Bulgur ⅔ cup - cooked	23
Corn flakes 1¼ cups	24
Couscous ⅔ cup - cooked	21
Muesli raw natural ⅔ cup	28
Noodles 1 cup - cooked	37
Oat bran raw 1 tbsp	7
Oatmeal 1 cup	25
Pearl barley ½ cup - cooked	22

Grains and Cereals	Carbohydrates (g)
Porridge ½ cup - cooked	45
Puffed wheat 1 cup	20
Rice basmati 1 cup - cooked	50
Rice bran 1 tbsp	5
Rice brown 1 cup - cooked	37
Rice instant 1 cup - cooked	37
Rice puffed 1 cup	11.5
Rice white 1 cup - cooked	50
Shredded wheat 1 cup	40
Special K 1 cup	22

Pasta - Cooked	Carbohydrates (g)
Cellophane noodles 1 cup	38
Fettuccini 1 cup	44
Gnocchi 1 cup	46
Macaroni 1 cup	40
Spaghetti white 60g	42
Spaghetti whole wheat 60g	40
Star pastina 1 cup	41
Vermicelli 1 cup	39

Breads	Carbohydrates (g)
Bagel 1	36
Bread crumbs 1 cup	73
Chapati (baisen flour) 1	25
Oat mix grain 1 slice	12
Pita 1 slice	33
Pumpernickel bread 1 slice	17
Rye 1 slice	15

Breads	Carbohydrates (g)
Sourdough 1 slice	21
White bread 1 slice	21
Whole-wheat 1 slice	15

Crackers	Carbohydrates (g)
Kavli 2	16
Rice cakes 3	123
Ryvita 2	16
Vita-weat sandwich size 3	25
Water crackers 3	18

Alcohol and Beverages	Carbohydrates (g)
Beer 1 can	13
Beer light 1 can	5
Coffee & tea no sugar	0
Coffee & tea with 2 tsp sugar	8.4
Cola 1 can	41
Gatorade 1 cup	14
Spirits 1½ oz (1 nip)	0
V8 veg. juice 1 cup	10
Wine 3 oz (1 glass)	3

Sugars	Carbohydrates (g)
Glucose 1tbsp	7.9
Honey 1 tbsp	8.2
Molasses 1 tbsp	5.5
Sugar - brown 1 tbsp	9.7
Sugar - white 1 tbsp	10

Animal protein (lean or fat)	Carbohydrates (g)
Fresh or canned fish, red meat, pork, poultry, eggs	1 to trace amounts
Clams raw & canned 90g	2
Crab meat canned 1 cup	2
Fish sticks, crumbed, frozen 4	16
Oysters ½ cup	4

Miscellaneous Items	Carbohydrates (g)
Black pepper 1 tsp	0.5
Cider vinegar 1 tbsp	1
Cinnamon 1 tsp	2
Curry powder 1 tsp	1
Garlic powder 1 tsp	2
Gherkin dill 1 medium	1
Gherkin sweet 1 medium	5
Jam - fruit 1 tbsp	18
Miso 1 oz	8
Mustard powder 1 tsp	trace
Onion powder 1 tsp	2
Oregano 1 tsp	1
Paprika 1 tsp	1
Relish or chutney 1 tbsp	5
Soup - tomato canned 1 cup	33
Tomato paste 1 cup	49
Tomato sauce 1 tbsp	2.5

Fast Food and Snack Food	Carbohydrates (g)
Cheese burger 1	28
Chocolate bar	69
Fish burger 1	39

Fast Food and Snack Food	Carbohydrates (g)
Fried chicken ½ breast	13
Hamburger 1	20
Jelly beans qty 10	10.3
Mars bar qty 53g	37.6
Oatmeal cookie with added sugar	54
Pizza 1 slice	39
Popcorn (popped - 1 cup)	5
Potato chips	51
Roast chicken ½ breast	0

Vegetables low in carbohydrates - Free foods
Alfalfa, asparagus, green beans, bamboo shoots, bean sprouts, cauliflower, cabbage, celery, collard greens, cucumber, dill pickle, eggplant, endive, fennel, kohlrabi, kale, lettuce, mushrooms, okra, onion up to 2 tbsp, parsley, bell peppers, radish, spinach, ½ tomato, turnips, zucchini and water cress.

Vegetable and fruit servings under 5 grams of carbohydrate for those on a low carbohydrate diet

Avocado ½ 8.5g
Blueberries 38g
Cabbage 90g
Asparagus 6 spears
Bell peppers ½ cup, chopped
Broccoli 1 cup, chopped
Brussels sprouts 4
Carrot 1
Cauliflower 1 cup, chopped
Chili pepper 1
Cucumber ½

Eggplant 30g
Green beans 45g
Leeks ½ cup
Mushrooms ½ cup
Parsley ½ cup, chopped
Shallots 1 tbsp
Spinach 60g
Strawberries 75g
Tomato ½ large
Waterchestnuts 4

Meats and nuts contain only tiny amounts of carbohydrate, or none at all. Their GI is close to zero, and if eaten alone, they have negligible effects on blood glucose levels.

Vegetable and Seed Oils
All have 0 to trace amounts of carbohydrates
Flaxseed, canola, olive, sunflower, coconut, grapeseed etc
Butter
Margarine
Note: The values above represent the average values taken from those in the scientific literature.

To search for Glycemic Index of foods

There is a website designed by the University of Sydney called www.glycemicindex.com which will enable you to calculate the Glycemic Index of common foods.

Food Labels

How to read and assess them

Have you ever been in the Supermarket or health food store and seen people pouring over food labels? I bet you have! It seems to have become of more interest to people today to read about what they are putting into their mouths. Then again you may have looked at these people and thought that they were eccentric – after all in the busy rush and tear of life who has time for that type of obsession?

Well it's really not that hard to understand a food label in a general way that will help you to make better food choices.

Become aware of what to look for on food labels. Avoid foods that have labels stating the presence of white flour, cornstarch, corn syrup, dextrose, maltose, sorbitol, aspartame, added sugar and hydrogenated vegetable oils.

Many supermarkets have health food sections, which are great to see, but even some so called health foods can be full of the bad fats and added sugar.

• Let us take a look at a basic food label – in this case it is from a brand of creamy peanut paste.

Creamy Peanut Butter (Brand A)	
Nutrition Facts Serving size 2 tbsp (32g) Servings per package 35	
Amount Per serving	
Calories 200 Calories from fat 140	
	% Daily value
Total Fat 16g	25%
Saturated fat 3g	15%
Cholesterol 0mg	0
Sodium 140mg	6%
Total Carbohydrate 6g	2%
Dietary fiber 2g	8%
Sugars 3g	
Protein 7g	
Ingredients: peanuts, sugar, hydrogenated vegetable oil (cotton seed & rapeseed), molasses, salt and diglycerides.	

The peanut butter Brand A is not recommended for your good health. How can you tell this from the label? The only clue is to read the ingredients, which states that it contains added sugar and hydrogenated vegetable oils. These are the oils you want to avoid, as they are processed oils laden with man made trans-fatty acids.

• Now let us take a look at the label from a healthy natural creamy peanut butter and see if you can spot the differences!

Creamy 100% Natural Peanut Butter (Brand B)	
Nutrition Facts Serving size 2 tbsp (32g) Servings about 14	
Amount Per serving	
Calories 200 Calories from fat 150	
	% Daily value
Total Fat 16g Saturated fat 2.5g **Cholesterol** 0mg **Sodium** 110mg **Total Carbohydrate** 7g Dietary fiber 2g Sugars 2g **Protein** 7g	25% 13% 0 5% 2% 9%
Ingredients: peanuts	

Comment: There are minor insignificant differences between the two Nutrition Facts panels, on Brand A and Brand B, which would not help you to decide which brand of peanut butter to buy. It is the ingredients list that will make the decision for you – in Brand B the only ingredients are real natural roasted peanuts and nothing else – there is no added sugar and no hydrogenated oils – in other words there is none of the unhealthy trans-fatty acids. So if you were switched on, you would buy Brand B and help your liver!

• Now let's compare 3 different brands of salad dressings, to find which is best for those with weight excess.

Creamy Salad Dressing (Brand A)	
Nutrition Facts Serving size 2 tbsp (1oz) Servings about 24	
Amount Per serving	
Calories 150 Calories from fat 140	
	% Daily value
Total Fat 16g	25%
Saturated fat 2.5g	13%
Cholesterol 10mg	3%
Sodium 290mg	12%
Total Carbohydrate 1g	0%
Dietary fiber 0g	0%
Sugars 1g	
Protein 0g	
Ingredients: hydrogenated soybean oil, sugar, vinegar, egg yolks, salt, skim milk, garlic juice, natural buttermilk flavor, monosodium glutamate, preservatives, spice, dried parsley, lemon juice concentrate & natural flavor.	

Raspberry Fat Free Salad Dressing (Brand B)	
Nutrition Facts Serving size 2 tbsp (1oz) Servings 8	
Amount Per serving	
Calories 35 Calories from fat 0	
	% Daily value
Total Fat 0g	0%
Saturated fat 0g	0%
Cholesterol 0mg	0%
Sodium 180mg	7%
Total Carbohydrate 9g	3%
Dietary fiber 0g	0%
Sugars 8g	
Protein 0g	
Ingredients: water, high fructose corn syrup, apple cider vinegar, cucumber juice, raspberry concentrate, lemon juice concentrate, salt, dehydrated red bell peppers, hibiscus fruit extract, citric acid, garlic powder, onion powder, xanthan gum, preservative, natural flavor.	

Extra Virgin Olive Oil Cold pressed (Brand C)	
Nutrition Facts Serving size 1 tbsp (½ oz) Servings about 66	
Amount Per serving	
Calories 120 Calories from fat 120	
	% Daily value
Total Fat 14g	22%
Saturated fat 2g	10%
Cholesterol 0mg	0%
Sodium 0mg	0%
Total Carbohydrate 0g	0%
Dietary fiber 0g	0%
Sugars 0g	
Protein 0g	
Ingredients: cold pressed virgin olive oil	

Comment:

Brand A of the salad dressing contains hydrogenated soybean oil, which contains unhealthy trans-fatty acids. It also contains added sugar and monosodium glutamate, which can cause headaches in some people.

Brand B of salad dressing is low in calories but contains a lot of added sugar from high fructose corn syrup. This will cause blood sugars to rise thus stimulating an increase in insulin levels.

Brand C of salad dressing is free of hydrogenated trans-fatty acids and is free of added sugar. It will have no effect upon blood glucose or insulin levels, and provides valuable mono-unsaturated fatty acids. Brand C is the preferred salad dressing for those with weight excess, and even at 240 calories per 2 tbsp, it is a superior dressing, as it is much healthier for the liver.

- Now let's look at the label of a very popular brand of breakfast cereal

Crunchy Wheat & Rice flakes with strawberries (Brand A) Fat Free!	
Nutrition Facts Serving size 1 cup (1.1oz) Servings about 11	
Amount Per serving	
Calories 110 Calories from fat 0	
	% Daily value
Total Fat 0g	0%
Saturated fat 0g	0%
Cholesterol 0mg	0%
Sodium 220mg	9%
Potassium 75mg	2%
Total Carbohydrate 25g	8%
Dietary fiber 1g	4%
Sugars 10g	
Other carbohydrates 14g	
Protein 4g	
Ingredients: rice, sugar, whole grain wheat, wheat gluten, freeze dried strawberries, defatted wheat germ, non-fat dried milk, high fructose corn syrup, salt, wheat flour, malt flavoring.	

Comment: Cereal Brand A may well be fat free, as they have stripped all the good fats from the wheat germ, and destroyed its vitamin E content in the process. You will note that its main ingredient is carbohydrate, which is in good part derived from refined sugar and refined high fructose corn syrup. This breakfast cereal is highly processed, and will cause a rapid rise in blood glucose, which is not the way to start your day if you have Syndrome X. You are better off to choose unrefined cereals, (such as unprocessed muesli) with no added sugar and no corn syrup. Then you will avoid the rapid rise in blood glucose after breakfast.

- Now lets look at some Premium chocolate chip cookies

Chocolate Chip Premium Cookies (Brand A)	
Nutrition Facts Serving size 1 cookie (1.24oz) Servings 26	
Amount Per serving	
Calories 150 Calories from fat 70	
	% Daily value
Total Fat 7g	11%
Saturated fat 4g	21%
Cholesterol 10mg	4%
Sodium 95mg	4%
Total Carbohydrate 22g	7%
Dietary fiber <1g	4%
Sugars 15g	
Protein 1g	
Ingredients: chocolate chips, bleached wheat flower, sugar, butter, margarine (partially hydrogenated vegetable oils from soybean & cottonseed) salt, diglycerides, artificial flavor, eggs, fructose, polydextrose, high fructose corn syrup, corn syrup, salt, baking soda, coconut oil, and numerous preservatives	

Comment: Brand A cookies are loaded with refined sugars and hydrogenated vegetable oils (trans-fatty acids). These things will send your blood glucose and insulin levels soaring.

The trans-fatty acids will be difficult for your liver to process and will adversely affect your blood fats.

I suggest that you try to find some healthier cookies free of added refined sugar and trans-fatty acids, or better still, avoid the cookies and eat fresh fruit and raw nuts.

Farewell Message

I do hope that you have enjoyed reading this book and that it has put the missing pieces of the jigsaw puzzle back together for you.

Writing this book has been a long journey for me. This book is the culmination of communicating with many thousands of overweight people via multiple means - face to face, by e-mail, in seminars and in my medical practice. I have talked to many weight loss experts and read their books and there was incredible divergence of opinion amongst the so-called experts. Some believed that the process of rapid fat burning, which leads to ketosis, was dangerous, whereas others thought it was the pathway to the Holy Grail of slimness. Amusingly I found that many of the experts were critical of each other's theories and books, but all held their own grains of truth amongst the confusion.

If you had time to read all of these books and websites, you would have a huge theoretical knowledge, but would probably be very confused. Furthermore you would not have any spare time to exercise!

I found that none of these books considered the liver as vitally important in the genesis of obesity. This oversight has always been astonishing to me, especially as today we are seeing an epidemic of fatty livers.

As always in life, if you live long enough, you come to the conclusion that you must tell your story the way you see it and understand it, in your own unique style. So I have tried to separate the wheat from the chaff, and present a balanced hybrid of modern day research and my own clinical experience.

Most of you will have tried many different diets and even weight loss surgery with varied success, but how many of you think that today in this present moment you are looking and feeling the best you can possibly be? According to current statistics not many of us!

You do not have to be overweight! You now have the knowledge, and thus the ability, to overcome the hormonal and metabolic problems that have been causing you to get fatter and fatter. It's not easy and it takes a lot of effort but this book gives you the vital clues and tools to fall back on. My strategy is holistic and makes you aware of all the causes that are keeping you trapped in the chemical imbalances, which lead to excess weight.

Weight Loss Detective Support

We are all individuals with unique hormonal, metabolic and psychological characteristics that need to be addressed for a successful long term outcome.

You can contact my Weight Loss Detectives with your questions if your weight loss is too slow or you are having problems following our metabolic weight loss plan.

Your weight loss detective can guide and support you by phone, skype and/or email correspondence. You can also have face to face consults if you live in an area close to a Weight Loss Detective.

Medical tests to pinpoint causes of weight gain include –

- Blood insulin and sugar (glucose) levels in the fasting state
- Blood leptin levels in the fasting state
- Saliva or blood levels for morning cortisol to check adrenal function
- Blood tests for gluten intolerant genes (HLA DQ genotype)
- Thyroid function (TSH, Free T 3, Reverse T 3), antibodies
- Liver enzymes
- Urine test for iodine concentration
- Stool analysis and PCR test for bacteria and parasites in the feces. Unhealthy micro-organisms in the gut can cause weight gain
- Salivary or blood tests for androgens and estrogens

You can email your results to a weight loss detective.

For further information call 623 334 3232 in the USA or 02 4655 8855 in Australia or email ehelp@liverdoctor.com

Stress, Depression and Anxiety

Stress can undo everything you are trying to achieve – and it will undo it quickly. Stress makes you lose your focus. To be successful you must be focused on yourself in a positive way – this is number one! You must work on your self esteem – you are worth it! I have a saying which is "Love Yourself to Health"

If you are addicted to food, stress will cause a drop in brain dopamine and blood sugar levels, and this will cause powerful cravings for your comfort food, or in other people cravings for alcohol or cigarettes etc.

Emotional eating may account for up to 80% of over eating. Emotional eating is dysfunctional and is the use of food to control negative emotions, anxiety or stress. The stress hormone (cortisol) also contributes directly to weight gain by increasing insulin resistance.

Hormonal Imbalances

These can be powerful causes of weight excess. The synthetic hormones in the contraceptive pill and many types of Hormone Replacement Therapy can lead to weight gain. Bio-identical hormones in the form of creams or capsules do not cause weight gain in m experience.

Pear shaped obesity or lower body weight gain in the buttocks, hips and thighs is found in Gynaeoid Body Types. This is associated with estrogen dominance and can be overcome with natural progesterone, the Body Type Supplements and the correct exercise program. There are many other causes of hormonal weight gain that may need to be addressed from Syndrome X, leptin resistance, excess androgens to thyroid resistance.

Food sensitivities and intolerances cause inflammation, which overworks the gut and liver leading to problems with metabolism. Food intolerances and allergies cause cravings, often for the very food that is causing the problem. The most common offenders are gluten and sugar.

The journey to your ideal weight goal can be difficult and may take longer then you anticipated. Take inspiration in the story of Dr Tom Eanelli MD, a medical specialist in New York who had a fatty liver and weighed 325 pounds. Dr Eanelli was successful with my program and now weighs 185 pounds and is fighting fit. He is grateful to me for saving his life; however he knows as a medical professional, just how hard it can be!

The stress can be high and your mind may try to fill you with negative thoughts that sabotage your efforts. Low self-esteem is at the root of most failures and causes us to give up - we may need help to maintain our self worth and confidence. It is not hopeless, as with our strategies you have a long-term plan that will work if you adopt it as a way of life. You do not have to be perfect and everyone needs little treats and comforts occasionally, especially if they feel empty and unloved. Remember that you need to "Love Yourself to Health."

You cannot fill up emptiness with chocolate, sugar, cigarettes, alcohol and carbohydrates. You can replace emptiness with a positive feeling that if you work on yourself to be the best you can possibly be, you will attract a fulfilling life. We are here to help you work on yourself by achieving what is possible through knowledge, science and compassion.

www.liverdoctor.com

www.drsandracabotclinics.com.au

www.sandracabot.com

My team and I are committed to your success - we are here to hold your hand and inspire you to reach a healthy weight and feel good about yourself!

Don't be shy - if you want more help and advice phone us on 623 334 3232 in the USA or 02 4655 8855 in Australia or E-mail Dr Cabot's naturopaths on ehelp@liverdoctor.com

References

Ref. 1. Reaven GM Pathophysiology of insulin resistance in human disease. Physiological Reviews. 1995;75(3):473-485.

Ref. 2. Assmann G, Schulte H. The importance of triglycerides: results from the Prospective Cardiovascular Muenster (PROCAM) Study. Eur J Epidemiol 1992; Supplement 1:99-103;

Assmann G.Schulte H. Relation of high-density lipoprotein cholesterol and triglycerides to incidence of atherosclerotic coronary artery disease (the PROCAM experience). Am J Cardiology 1992; 70:733-37.

Ref. 3. Reissell P K et al. Treatment of hypertriglyceridemia. Am J Clin Nutr 1966; 19:84 - 98.

Ref. 4. Sanchez - Delgado E, Liechti H. Lifetime risk of developing coronary heart disease. Lancet 1999; 353:934.

Ref. 5. U.S. Bureau of Census.

Ref. 6. Smith M A et al. Advanced Maillard reaction end products are associated with Alzheimer disease pathology. Proc Nat Acad Sci USA 1994; 91:5710 - 14 and Vitek M P et al. Advanced glycation end products contribute to amyloidosis in Alzheimer disease Proc Nat Acad Sci USA 1994; 91: 4766 - 70.

Ref. 7. - Gymnema Sylvestre

Use of Gymnema Sylvestre Leaf Extract in the control of blood glucose in insulin-dependent diabetes mellitus, Shanmugasundaram. G et al. Dept. Biochemistry, University of Madras, Madras 600-113, Elsevier Scientific Publishers Ireland 1990

Studies on the Hypoglycemic Action of Gymnema Sylvestre, Dept. Biochemistry, University of Madras 600 042, Arogya -J. Health Sci., 1981, VII, 38-60.

Antidiabetic Effect of a leaf extract from Gymnema Sylvestre in non-insulin dependent diabetes mellitus patients, K. Baskaran et al. Journal of Ethnopharmacology, 30(1990) 295-305, Elsevier Scientific Publishers Ireland Ltd.

Ref. 8. - Momordica charantia (Bitter Melon)

Leatherdale, B.A. et al. Improvement in glucose tolerance due to Momordica charantia, (1981) British Medical Journal, 282: 1823-1824.

Sarkar, S. et al. Demonstration of the Hypoglycemic action of Momordica charantia in a validated animal model of diabetes. 1996 Pharmacological Research, 33(1):1-4.

Akhtar M.S. (1982) Trial of Momordica charantia powder in patients with maturity onset diabetes. Journal of the Pakistan Medical Association. 32:106-107

Welihinda, J. et al. Effect of Momordica charantia on the glucose tolerance in maturity onset diabetes.1986, J. Ethnopharmacology 17:277-282 Cunnick J. 1993, Bitter Melon, Journal of Naturopathic Medicine. 4(1): 261

Ref. 9 & 10. - Chromium

Kaats g et al. Effects of chromium picolinate on body composition. A randomized double-masked, placebo-controlled study. Current Therap. Research (1996) 57(10):747-765

Anderson RA et al. Elevated intakes of supplemental chromium improve glucose and insulin variables in individuals with type II diabetes. Diabetes (1997);46:1786-91

Cunningham JJ. Micronutrients as nutraceutical interventions in diabetes mellitus. J. Am Coll Nutr. 1998;17(1):7-10

References

Ref. 11. - Lipoic Acid

Sachse G & Willms B. Efficiency of thioctic acid (lipoic acid) in the therapy of peripheral diabetic neuropathy. Hormone & Metabolic Research (Supplement). 9:105, 1980

Wagh SS et al. Mode of action of lipoic acid in diabetes. Journal of Bioscience. 11:59-74, 1987. Chromium Picolinate Liu, V. J.,

Chromium & Insulin in young subjects with normal glucose tolerance. Am. J. Clin. Nutr. 25(4) 1982, pp. 661-667

Jacob S. et al. Enhancement of glucose disposal in patients with type 2 diabetes by alpha-lipoic acid. Arzneim - Rorsch Drug Res. 1995;45(2):872-874

Jacob S. et al. The antioxidant alpha-lipoic acid enhances insulin-stimulated glucose metabolism in insulin-resistant rat skeletal muscle. Diabetes. 1996;45:1024-1029

Jacobs et al. Enhancement of glucose disposal in patients with type 11 diabetes by alpha-lipoic acid. Arzneimittel-Forschung (1993) 45:87274

Strodter D et al. The influence of lipoic acid (thioctic acid) on metabolism and function of the diabetic heart. Diabetic Res. Clin. Prac. (1995) 29(1):19-26

Packer L et al. Neuro protection by the metabolic antioxidant alpha lipoic acid. Free Radical Biol. Med. (1997) 22(1-2): 359-78

Khamaisis M: Lipoic acid reduces glycemia and increases muscle GLUT 4 content in diabetic rats. Metabolism 46(7), 763-768 (1997)

Jacob S; The antioxidant alpha-lipoic acid enhances insulin-stimulated glucose metabolism in insulin-resistant rat skeletal muscle. Diabetes 45(8), 1024-1029 (1996)

Ziegler D et al. (1997) Alpha-lipoic acid in the treatment of diabetic peripheral and cardiac autonomic neuropathy. Diabetes 46 (Suppl 2): S62-S66

Ref. 12. - Carnitine

Pola P. et al. Carnitine in the therapy of dyslipidemic patients. Curr. Ther. Res. 27:208 - 216, 1980

Rebouche CJ and Engel AG. Carnitine metabolism & Deficiency Syndromes. Mayo Clinic Proceedings. 58:533 - 540, 1983

Rossi CS & Siliprandi N. Effect of carnitine on serum HDL-cholesterol: report of cases. John Hopkins Medical Journal. 150:51-54, 1982

Ref. 13. - Selenium Margaret Rayman, "Dietary Selenium; time to act", British Medical Journal, Vol. 314, 387, Feb 1997

Ref. 14. - Zinc

Solomon, S.J. et al, Effect of low zinc intake on carbohydrate & fat metabolism in men. Federal Proc. 42 (1983), p.391.

Tauri, S. Studies of zinc metabolism: Effect of the diabetic state on zinc metabolism: A clinical aspect. Endocrinology Japan 10 (1963), pp. 9-15

Faure P. et al. Zinc prevents the structural and functional properties of free radical treated-insulin. Biochimica et Biophysica Acta. 1994;1209:260-264

Ref. 15. - Silymarin (St Mary's Thistle)

Boari C, et al, Occupational toxic liver diseases. Therapeutic effects of Silymarin. Min Med 1985; 72(2):679-88

Flora K, et al. Milk Thistle (Silybum marianum) for the therapy of liver disease. Am. J. Gastroenterol 1998 Feb; 93(2): 139-43

Salmi HA, et al, Effect of silymarin on chemical, functional and morphological alteration of the liver: a double blind controlled study. Scandinavian J. Gastroenterology 1982; 17:417-21

Ref. 16. - Taurine

Orthoplex Research Bulletin, Taurine the detoxifying amino acid. Nutrients in profile, Henry Osiecki. Bioconcepts Publishing

Ref. 17. - Globe Artichoke S. Rocchietta, Minerva Med. 50, 612, 1959)

Parveen J. Kumar BSc. MD, FRCP, Clinical Medicine, Liver Function, page 237-287, Bailliere Tindall

Ref. 19. -Bland J.S., Bralley J.A. Nutritional up-regulation of hepatic detoxification enzymes. The Journal of Applied Nutrition, 1992,44; No. 3 & 4

Cabre E, et al. Nutritional Support in liver disease. Eur J Gastroenterol Hepatol 1995;7(6): 528-32

Meister A. Selective modification of glutathione metabolism. Science 220:472-477, 1983,

The Doctor's Vitamin Encyclopedia, Arrow Books, Dr Sheldon Hendler. M.D., Stevia

Jeppesen PB, et al. Stevioside acts directly on pancreatic beta cells to secrete insulin. Metabolism 2000 Feb;49(2):208-14

Akashi, J. and Yokohama. Safety of extract of dried stevia leaves results of toxicity tests. Shokuhin Kogya, 10B:34-43, 1975

Bridel M. and Lavielle. Le principe a saveur sucree du Kaa-he-e (Stevia rebaudiana Bertoni). J. Pharm. Clin, 14:99-154, 1931

Kinghorn A.D. et al. Current status of stevioside as a sweetening agent for human use. Economic and Medicinal Plant Research, London: Academic Press, Inc., 1985

Ishii- Iwamoto et al. Stevioside is not metabolized in the isolated perfused rat liver. Research Communications in Molecular Pathology & Pharmacology, 87:167-175, 1995

Crammer B. and R. Ikan, Progress in the chemistry and properties of stevia rebaudioside. Developments in Sweeteners. London, Elsevier, vol. 3:45-64, 1987

Fletcher, Hewitt, Jr. The sweet herb of Paraguay. Chemurgic Digest, 18, July/August, 1955

Olney J. W., N.B. Farber et al. Increasing brain tumor rates: is there a link to aspartame? Journal of Neuropathology & Experimental Neurology, 55(11):1115-1123, 1996

Ref. 23. Suttajit M. et al. Mutagenicity and human chromosomal effects of stevioside, a sweetener from stevia rebaudiana. Environmental Health Perspectives Supplement, 101 (3):53-56, 1993.

Ref. 24 & 25. Curi, R., M. Alvarez, et al. Effect of stevia rebaudiana on glucose tolerance in normal adult humans. Brazilian Journal of Medicine & Biological Research, 19(6):771-774, 1986

Alvarez M. et al. Effect of aqueous extract of stevia rebaudiani on biochemical parameters of normal adult persons. Arq. Biol. Tech, 24:178, 1981

Nunes, P., N.A. Pereira. The effect of stevia rebaudiana on the fertility of experimental animals. Revista Brasileira de Farmacia, 69:46-50, 1988

Klongpanichpak, S., et al. lack of mutagenicity of stevioside and steviol in Salmonella typhimurium TA 98 & TA 100. Journal Medical Associations of Thailand, Sep; 80, Suppl 1:S121-128, 1997

Ref. 26. Melis, M.S. A crude extract of Stevia rebaudiana increases the renal plasma flow of normal and hypertensive rats. Brazilian Journal of Medicine & Biological Research, 29(5):660-675, 1996

Yodyingyaud, V. et al. Effect of Stevioside on growth and reproduction. Human Reproduction,

References

6(1):158-165, 1991

Toyada K. et al. Assessment of the carcinogenicity of stevioside in F344 rats. Food & Chemical Toxicology, 35(6):597-603, 1997

Xili, L. et al. Chronic oral toxicity and carcinogenicity study of stevioside in rats. Food Chemistry Toxicology, 30:957-965, 1992

Von Schmelling, G.A., et al. Stevia rebaudiani : Evaluation of the Hypoglycemic effect in alloxanized rabbits. Ciencia e Cultura, 29(5):599-601, 1977

Ref. 28. Dreon D M, et al. A very low-fat diet is not associated with improved lipoprotein profiles in men with a predominance of large, low-density lipoproteins. Am J Clin Nutr 1999; 69:411-18

Ref. 30. Barnard D E et al. Dietary Trans-fatty acids modulate erythrocyte membrane fatty acyl composition and insulin binding in monkeys. J Nutr Biochem 1990; 1:190-95;

Kuller L H. Trans-fatty acids and dieting (letter). Lancet 1993; 341:1093-94

Mann G V. Metabolic consequences of dietary Trans-fatty acids. Lancet 1994; 343:1268-71

Ref. 31.

Willett W C, et al. Intake of Trans-fatty acids on risk of coronary heart disease among women. Lancet 1993; 341:581-85

Ref. 32. Glutamine

Ballard T. et al. Effect of Glutamine Supplementation on impaired glucose regulation during intravenous lipid administration. Dept. of Surgery, Duke University Medical Center and Veterans Affairs Medical Center, Durham, North Carolina, USA. Nutrition 1996;12:349-354

Ref. 33. Glucagon

Muller, W. A. et al. The Influence of the antecedent diet upon glucagon and insulin secretion. New England Journal of Medicine 285 (1971), pp. 1450 - 1454.

Diabetes

Reaven P. Dietary & pharmacological regimes to reduce lipid peroxidation in non-insulin-dependent diabetes mellitus. Am. J. Clin. Nutr. 1995;62:1483S-1489S

Thompson KH. Et al. Micronutrients and antioxidants in the progression of diabetes. Nutrition Research 1995;15(9):1377-1410

Schleicher E. et al. Increased accumulation of the glycoxidation product N (epsilon) - (carboxymethyl) lysien in human tissues in diabetes and ageing. Journal of Clinical Investigations, 99:457-468, 1997

Klok MD, Jakobsdottir S, Drent ML. The role of leptin and ghrelin in the regulation of food intake and body weight in humans: a review. Obes Rev. 2007 Jan;8(1):21-34. Review.

Woods SC. The control of food intake: behavioral versus molecular perspectives. Cell Metab. 2009 Jun;9(6):489-98. Review.

Shapiro A, et al. Fructose-induced leptin resistance exacerbates weight gain in response to subsequent high-fat feeding. Am. J. Physiol. Regul. Integr. Comp. Physiol. 2008. 295 (5): R1370–5.

Münzberg H, Flier JS, Bjørbaek C. Region-specific leptin resistance within the hypothalamus of diet-induced obese mice. Endocrinology. 2004 Nov;145(11):4880-9.

Inui A. Ghrelin: an orexigenic and somatotrophic signal from the stomach. Nat Rev Neurosci. 2001 Aug;2(8):551-60. Review.

Barkan, et al. Ghrelin secretion in humans is sexually dimorphic, suppressed by somatostatin, and not affected by the ambient growth hormone levels. The Journal of Clinical Endocrinology

& Metabolism Vol. 88, No. 5 2180-2184. doi:10.1210/jc.2002-021169

Ramel A, et al. Beneficial effects of long-chain n-3 fatty acids included in an energy-restricted diet on insulin resistance in overweight and obese European young adults. Diabetologia. 2008 Jul;51(7):1261-8. Epub 2008 May 20.

Pejovic S, et al. Leptin and hunger levels in young healthy adults after one night of sleep loss. J Sleep Res. 2010 Dec;19(4):552-8

Taheri S, et al. Short Sleep Duration Is Associated with Reduced Leptin, Elevated Ghrelin, and Increased Body Mass Index. 2004. PLoS Med 1(3):e62

Greaves CJ, et al. Systematic review of reviews of intervention components associated with increased effectiveness in dietary and physical activity interventions. BMC Public Health. 2011 Feb 18;11(1):119.

AACE Medical Guidelines for Clinical Practice for the Evaluation and Treatment of Hyperthyroidism and Hypothyroidism, Endocrine Practice, Vol. 8, No. 6, Nov/Dec 2002.